Clinical Vision Science

Gunnar Schmidtmann

Clinical Vision Science

A Concise Guide to Numbers, Laws, and Formulas

Second Edition 2025

Springer

Gunnar Schmidtmann
School of Health Professions
University of Plymouth
Plymouth, UK

ISBN 978-3-031-83320-5 ISBN 978-3-031-83321-2 (eBook)
https://doi.org/10.1007/978-3-031-83321-2

This Springer imprint is published by the registered company Springer Nature Switzerland AG
The registered company address is: Gewerbestrasse 11, 6330 Cham, Switzerland

*This book is dedicated to my parents Sylvia and Wolfgang,
and my family Fiona and Roselyn.*

Preface

Students, trainees, and clinicians in optometry, ophthalmology and related subjects are often confronted with many numbers, units, and procedures to memorize and recall during their studies, for exam preparations and in practice. A small handbook that fits into a lab coat pocket would be the ideal resource to refresh the knowledge quickly. This handbook serves as a quick guide for the most important facts, numbers, laws and clinical procedures for students and clinicians in the clinical vision sciences. It is aimed at students and trainees in optometry, orthoptics, ophthalmology and vision science.

This handbook is composed of short chapters covering many relevant domains ranging from physical optics to anatomy and clinical procedures. Each chapter contains concisely summarized and visualized key concepts, formulas with descriptions, clear tables, custom-made illustrations and flow charts designed to demonstrate complex concepts comprehensively. Particularly important facts are highlighted in distinct boxes. This second, completely revised edition also contains exercises at the end of each chapter. The answers and solutions are provided in a separate new chapter at the end of the book. It is important to emphasize that this handbook does not replace a textbook in any of the covered topics. Hence, a list of further readings is provided at the end of each chapter.

Plymouth, UK
September 2024

Gunnar Schmidtmann

Acknowledgements

I would like to thank the students at the University of Plymouth who inspired me to write this book and who provided useful feedback. I am particularly grateful to my colleague and friend Paul Artes for his support and encouragement. I also want to acknowledge my colleagues Hetal and Phillip Buckhurst, whose lectures on Physical and Physiological Optics inspired the content of this handbook. Finally, I would like to thank Sae Bom Ra from Adelphi University, and Samantha Strong from Aston University for the beautiful anatomical illustrations in Chap. 9.

Contents

List of Figures

List of Tables

1

Basics

A good understanding of fundamental mathematical concepts is essential to understand physical and visual optics. This chapter seeks to introduce some basic mathematical and physical principles, symbols, units, calculations, and conversions that will be useful throughout your studies and beyond. Test your knowledge with the exercises provided at the end of this chapter.

1.1 Greek Alphabet

The Greek alphabet has been extensively used in science, mathematics, and various other academic disciplines for centuries. Its letters are often used as symbols to represent mathematical constants, variables, functions, and other quantities. The lower–and upper-case letters of the Greek alphabet are shown in Table 1.1.

G. Schmidtmann, *Clinical Vision Science*,
https://doi.org/10.1007/978-3-031-83321-2_1

Table 1.1 The Greek alphabet

α A	Alpha	ι I	Iota	ρ ϱ P	Rho
β B	Beta	κ K	Kappa	σ Σ	Sigma
γ Γ	Gamma	λ Λ	Lambda	τ T	Tau
δ Δ	Delta	μ M	Mu	υ Υ	Upsilon
ϵ ε E	Epsilon	ν N	Nu	ϕ φ Φ	Phi
ζ Z	Zeta	ξ Ξ	Xi	χ X	Chi
η H	Eta	o O	Omicron	ψ Ψ	Psi
θ ϑ Θ	Theta	π Π	Pi	ω Ω	Omega

1.2 Angular Measures

Figure 1.1 shows a circle with a radius of 1 unit centered at the origin (0,0) in a Cartesian coordinate system. This is referred to as the unit circle, which is a fundamental concept in trigonometry and geometry. The angle θ denotes the central angle (shown here at 45°). The angle θ can be expressed in degrees and describes the fraction of a complete revolution around the circle, where one complete revolution corresponds to 360°. Hence, an angle of 90° corresponds to a quarter, and 180° to half of the circumference, respectively.

However, angles can also be expressed in radians. In the context of the unit circle, an angle measured in radians is defined as the length of the corresponding arc along the unit circle divided by the radius of the circle. Since the radius of the unit circle is 1 unit, an angle of 1 radian would correspond to an arc length equal to the radius. Similarly, an angle of π radian ($\pi \approx 3.14159$) would correspond to halfway the circumference of the circle, because π radians is half the circumference of the unit circle. A full revolution around the unit circle corresponds to $2 \cdot \pi$ radians. This is relevant for the trigonometric functions (see Sect. 1.4).

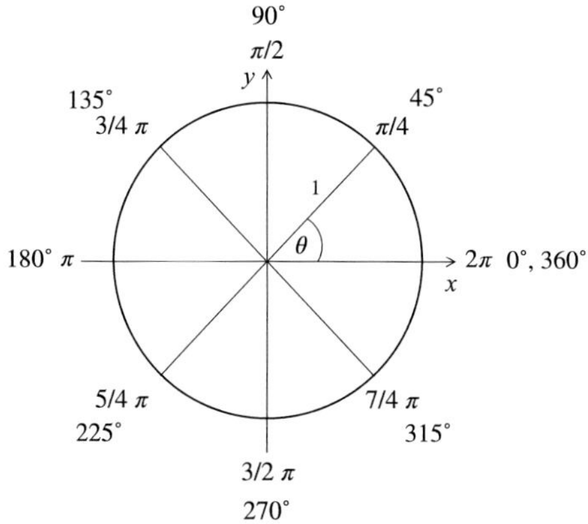

Fig. 1.1 The unit circle with angles defined in degrees and radians

Given the abovementioned relationship between degrees and radians, one can easily convert degrees to radians and vice versa. The relevant equations are shown below.

1.2.1 Degrees to Radians

$$\alpha_{Radians} = \frac{\alpha_{Degree} \cdot \pi}{180^{\circ}} \tag{1.1}$$

1.2.2 Radians to Degree

$$\alpha_{Degree} = \frac{\alpha_{Radians} \cdot 180^{\circ}}{\pi} \tag{1.2}$$

1.2.3 Degree, Arc Minute and Arc Second

We often deal with very small angles (e.g., the visual angle in visual acuity measurements). It is convenient to express

very small angles in arc minutes (arc min, $'$) or arc seconds (arc sec, $''$), instead of fractions of degrees ($^\circ$).
$1^\circ = 60'$ [arc min]
$1' = 60''$ [arc sec]

1.3 Pythagorean Theorem

Pythagoras' or Pythagorean theorem is a fundamental principle in geometry that relates to right (right-angled) triangles. It states that in a right triangle, the square of the length of the hypotenuse (the side opposite the right angle) is equal to the sum of the squares of the lengths of the other two sides (legs). Pythagorean theorem is illustrated in Fig. 1.2. The figure shows a right triangle, where the side a denotes the opposite, b the adjacent, and c the hypotenuse. The squares illustrate the mathematical operation of squaring each side (i.e., a^2, b^2, c^2)

$$a^2 + b^2 = c^2 \tag{1.3}$$

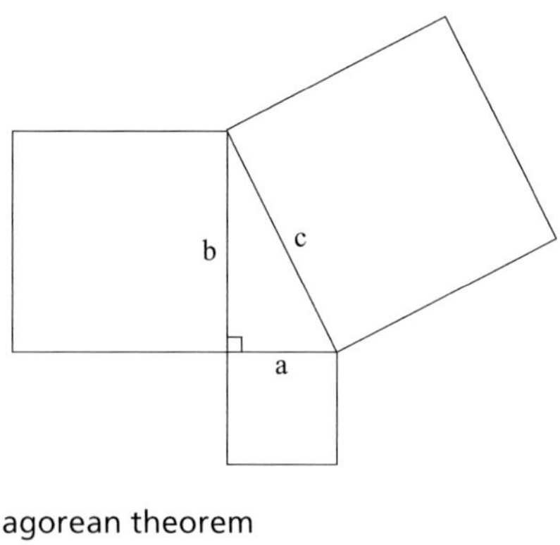

Fig. 1.2 Pythagorean theorem

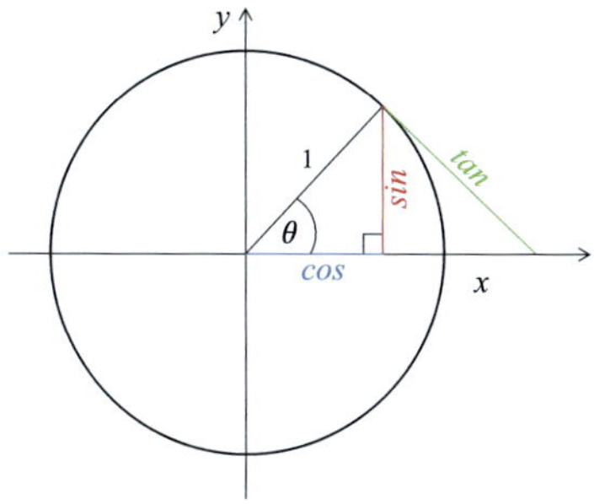

Fig. 1.3 The unit circle with the main trigonometric functions

1.4 Trigonometry

Figure 1.3 shows a unit circle with the most important trigonometric functions of θ, where sin refers to the sine (red), cos to the cosine (blue), and tan to the tangent (green) of θ.

1.4.1 Trigonometric Functions

Figure 1.4 shows a right triangle $\triangle ABC$, where the side a denotes the opposite, b the adjacent, and c the hypotenuse. Trigonometric functions are mathematical functions that relate the angles of a right triangle to the lengths of its sides.

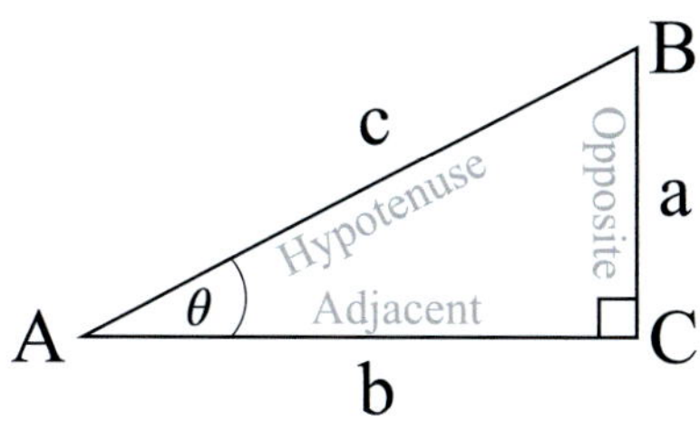

Fig. 1.4 Right triangle $\triangle ABC$ with labeling of vertices and sides

$$\sin\theta = \frac{a}{c} \tag{1.4}$$

$$\cos\theta = \frac{b}{c} \tag{1.5}$$

$$\tan\theta = \frac{a}{b} \tag{1.6}$$

1.4.1.1 The Sine and Cosine Functions

So far we have defined the trigonometric functions by using the unit circle, but we can also define these functions in a Cartesian[1] coordinate system, where the general form of a sine function is given by:

$$y = A \cdot sin(x \cdot \omega + \varphi) \tag{1.7}$$

where A denotes the amplitude, ω the frequency, and φ the phase or period. Changes in A, ω, and φ are illustrated in Fig. 1.5.

1.4.2 Inverse Trigonometric Functions

For certain calculations one requires the inverse of the trigonometric functions. The most relevant functions are shown below.

$$\arcsin x = \sin^{-1} x \tag{1.8}$$

$$\arccos x = \cos^{-1} x \tag{1.9}$$

$$\arctan x = \tan^{-1} x \tag{1.10}$$

[1]The term Cartesian refers to the French mathematician and philosopher René Descartes (1596–1650).

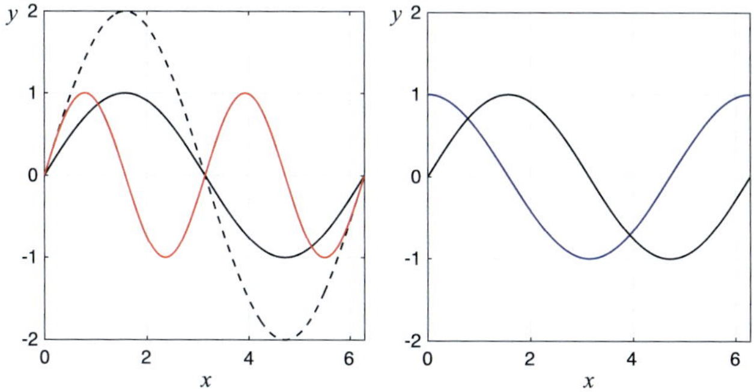

Fig. 1.5 The black solid line in the left graph shows a basic sine function with an amplitude $A = 1$, frequency $\omega = 1$, and phase (period) $\varphi = 0$. The dashed black line shows the same sine function with an amplitude $A = 2$. The red solid line shows the influence of the frequency ω, which was increased to $\omega = 2$. The black solid line in the right graph shows the basic sine function. The blue function illustrates a change of the phase by $\varphi = \pi/2$. Note that the phase shift of $\varphi = \pi/2$ changes the sine function into a cosine function (see Fig. 1.3 to undertand the relationship beween sine and cosine)

1.5 Exponentiation and Logarithms

1.5.1 Exponentiation

In order to understand logarithms, we first have to understand the concept of exponentiation. Exponentiation is a mathematical operation that involves raising a base number b to a certain power, known as an exponent y. The result of exponentiation is the base number multiplied by itself a certain number of times, determined by the value of the exponent y.

$$b^y = x \tag{1.11}$$

Logarithms are mathematical functions that represent the inverse operations of exponentiation. In simpler terms, logarithms answer the question "To what power must a given base be raised to produce a given number?". Hence, the logarithm of a number x to a specified base b is denoted as:

$$y = \log_b(x) \tag{1.12}$$

which is read as: y is the logarithm of x to the base b.

Logarithms are a very useful mathematical concept with countless applications in many fields, including mathematics, engineering, and physics. With respect to the vision sciences, logarithms are important to understand the progression of letter optotypes on common visual acuity charts (e.g., the Bailey-Lovie or logMAR chart [1]), or the decibel (dB) unit of changes in light intensity used in perimetry (see Sect. 1.8.1).

The notation log typically refers to a logarithm to the base 10, whereas ln refers to the logarithm to the base of the number e (natural logarithm), where e is Euler's number.[2]

The number e is the limit

$$\lim_{n\to\infty}\left(1+\frac{1}{n}\right)^n, \tag{1.13}$$

and can be exressed as the sum of the infinite series

$$e = \sum_{n=0}^{\infty}\frac{1}{n!} = \frac{1}{1}+\frac{1}{1}+\frac{1}{1\cdot 2}+\frac{1}{1\cdot 2\cdot 3}+\ldots = 2.71828\ldots \tag{1.14}$$

$$\log_e(x) = \ln(x) \tag{1.15}$$

[2] Euler's number is a mathematical constant named after the mathematician Leonhard Euler (1707–1783).

1.5.2 Calculation Rules

$$\log_a(x \cdot y) = \log_a(x) + \log_a(y)$$

$$\log_a\left(\frac{x}{y}\right) = \log_a(x) - \log_a(y)$$

$$\log_a(x^c) = c \cdot \log_a(x)$$

1.6 The Metric System

The metric system is a systematic decimal-based system of measurement. It was developed as a standardized and rational system of measurement to replace the diverse and often confusing array of measurement systems used in different regions and applications. The metric system is characterized by its use of decimal multiples and submultiples of basic units, making conversions between units straightforward. The metric system has been widely adopted around the world due to its simplicity, ease of use, and compatibility with scientific notation. It is used in many countries as the official system of measurement for commerce, industry, education, and scientific research. In addition to the base units, the metric system also includes prefixes to denote multiples and submultiples of units, such as kilo- (10^3), centi- (10^{-2}), and milli- (10^{-3}). Table 1.2 summarizes the most important prefixes.

Table 1.2 The metric system

Prefix	Symbol	Power	Factor
Exa	E	10^{18}	1,000,000,000,000,000,000
Peta	P	10^{15}	1,000,000,000,000,000
Tera	T	10^{12}	1,000,000,000,000
Giga	G	10^{9}	1,000,000,000
Mega	M	10^{6}	1,000,000
Kilo	k	10^{3}	1,000
Hecto	h	10^{2}	100
Deca	da	10^{1}	10
Non	non	10^{0}	1
Deci	d	10^{-1}	0.1
Centi	c	10^{-2}	0.01
Milli	m	10^{-3}	0.001
Micro	μ	10^{-6}	0.000,001
Nano	n	10^{-9}	0.000,000,001
Pico	p	10^{-12}	0.000,000,000,001
Femto	f	10^{-15}	0.000,000,000,000,001
Atto	A	10^{-18}	0.000,000,000,000,000,001

1.7 International System of Units

The SI units (International System of Units) are a standard system of measurement used in science, engineering, and everyday life. They provide a consistent and internationally recognized set of units for expressing physical quantities. The SI system is based on seven base units, from which all other units are derived. These base units are shown in Table 1.3.

Table 1.3 International system of units

Unit name	Unit symbol	Dimension symbol	Quantity name
Metre	m	L	Length
Kilogram	kg	M	Mass
Second	s	T	Time
Ampere	A	I	Electric current
Kelvin	K	Θ	Thermodynamic temperature
Mole	mol	N	Amount of substance
Candela	cd	J	Luminous intensity

1.8 Important Physical Units

Optometry and ophthalmology, and vision science in general, rely heavily on accurate measurements of various physical quantities such as distance, size, refractive power, light intensity, and many more. Physical units serve as the language through which practitioners communicate, ensuring consistency and clarity in diagnoses and treatment. Whether it is measuring visual acuity, quantifying intraocular pressure in Millimetres of Mercury ($mmHg$), or assessing the curvature of the cornea in diopters (D), each unit carries vital information essential for understanding ocular health and functionality. It is therefore important to have a basic understanding of some common physical units. Some of the most important units, their symbols, and derived units, and their relationship to each other, are summarized in Table 1.4.

Table 1.4 Important units

Quantity	Name	Symbol	Derived unit
Frequency	Hertz	Hz	$\frac{1}{s} = s^{-1}$
Force	Newton	N	$\frac{kg \cdot m}{s^2}$
Energy	Joule	J	$N \cdot m = \frac{kg \cdot m^2}{s^2}$
Power	Watt	W	$\frac{J}{s} = \frac{kg \cdot m^2}{s^3}$
Pressure	Pascal	Pa	$\frac{N}{m^2} = \frac{kg}{m \cdot s^2}$
Luminous flux	Lumen	lm	$cd \cdot sr$
Illumination	Lux	lx	$\frac{cd \cdot sr}{m^2}$

1.8.1 Decibel

The decibel (dB) is a logarithmic unit used to express the ratio between two quantities I_1 and I_2 (typically power or intensity) on a logarithmic scale. This unit is commonly used in fields such as acoustics, electronics, telecommunications, signal processing, but also perimetry (visual fields) to describe the relative level of light, sound, electrical signals, or other quantities. For instance, in standard perimetry the sensitivity to light is measured in decibels.

$$10 \cdot \log\left(\frac{I_2}{I_1}\right) \text{dB} \tag{1.16}$$

I_1: Intensity

I_2: Reference intensity

Example

$I_1 = 10$

$I_2 = 10,000$

$$10 \cdot \log\left(\frac{10,000}{10}\right) = 30 \text{ dB}$$

1.8.2 Pressure

The unit pressure (P) refers to the amount of force (F) applied per unit area (A). It is typically measured in units such as Pascal (SI unit, Pa), pounds per square inch (psi), atmospheres (atm), or bars (bar), depending on the system of measurement being used.

Mathematically, the pressure can be expressed as:

$$P = \frac{F}{A} \tag{1.17}$$

F: Force

A: Area

Clinically, the pressure is frequently measured in the unit Millimetre of Mercury ($mmHg$). This unit of pressure is commonly used in the measurment of blood pressure, and also the intraocular pressure.

Conversion

$1\ mmHg = \ 133.322 Pa$

$1\ Pa = \ 7.5 \cdot 10^{-3} mmHg$

1.9 Exercises

Note that all exercises below can be solved without the use of a calculator.

1. Convert the angle $\beta = 90°$ to radians.
2. Convert the angle $\gamma = 2 \cdot \pi$ (radians) to degrees.

3. The hypothenuse of a right triangle has a lenght of $\sqrt{2}$, and the opposite has a length of 1. What is the length of the adjacent?
4. What is the solution of $log_{10}10,000$?
5. Rearrange $x = 2 \cdot e^{4y^2}$ to make y the subject.
6. The Force F is calculated according to the equation $F = m \cdot a$, where m is the mass measured in kg and a is the acceleration measured in $^m/_{s^2}$. Derive the SI unit of the Force F? Hint: Newton is not the answer we are looking for!

1.10 Further Reading

- Tunnacliffe AH. Introduction to visual optics. London: Association of british dispensing opticians; 1993.
- Tunnacliffe AH., Hirst, JG., Optics. Association of British Dispensing Opticians. London; 1996.
- Weltner K., Grosjean J., Weber WJ., Schuster P., Mathematics for Physicist and Engineers. Springer; 2009.
- Whitehead, AN. An introduction to mathematics. Courier Dover Publications; 2017.

Reference

1. Bailey IL, Lovie JE. New design principles for visual acuity letter charts. Optomet Vis Sci. 1976;53(11):740–5.

2

Physical Optics

The term optics refers to the branch of physics dedicated to the science of light. The manipulation of light is at the heart of optics and optometric and ophthalmic practice. For instance, reflection and refraction are the physical principles that can be utilized to reflect and focus light in spectacles, contact lenses and optical instruments.

In this chapter, I will introduce the most important concepts of geometrical and physical optics. After a brief introduction to the properties of light, I will cover the basics of refraction and reflection. A basic knowledge of geometrical optics will help you to develop an understanding of how mirrors, prisms and lenses can be used to direct light.

2.1 Nature of Light

The term light refers to the entire spectrum of the electromagnetic radiation, ranging from γ-Rays to long radio waves (see Fig. 2.1). The electromagnetic radiation can be imag-

G. Schmidtmann, *Clinical Vision Science*,
https://doi.org/10.1007/978-3-031-83321-2_2

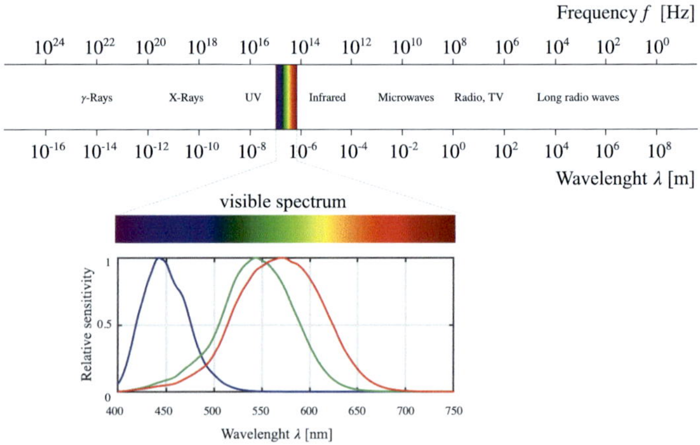

Fig. 2.1 The figure shows an illustration of the electromagnetic spectrum. The top panel shows the various types of the electromagnetic radiation characterized by their frequency f measured in Hz, and wavelength λ in m. The middle panel shows an enlarged version of the visible spectrum (i.e. visible light) with the corresponding perceived colors and wavelengths λ in nm. The bottom panel shows the relative spectral sensitivities of the human cone photoreceptors, specifically short (S, blue), medium (M, green), and long (L, red) wavelength cones [1–3]

ined as a wave with a specific wavelentgh λ (often expressed in nm), and frequency f [$^1/_s = Hz$]. The wavelength λ and frequency f are inversely proportional, i.e. the wavelength increases as the frequency decreases, and vice versa. The relationship between λ and f is:

$$f = \frac{v}{\lambda} \tag{2.1}$$

v: Velocity [$^m/_s = ms^{-1}$]
f: Frequency [$^1/_s = s^{-1} = Hz$]
λ: Wavelength [m]

In vacuum, the electromagnetic waves travel at the speed of light c. In this special case $v = c$, hence:

$$f = \frac{c}{\lambda} \tag{2.2}$$

Light that can be perceived by humans is called visible light or visible spectrum with wavelengths ranging from around 380 to 700 nm [4].

Light has both, wave and particle characteristics. The particle of light is called photon, which has an energy E that is proportional to its frequency f, by:

$$E = h \cdot f = \frac{h \cdot c}{\lambda} \tag{2.3}$$

E: Photon Energy
h: Planck's constant[1] ($6.626070040 \cdot 10^{34} J \cdot s$)
c: Speed of light (299,792,458 m/s)

2.2 Refraction

2.2.1 Refractive Index

The speed of light c depends on the medium (i.e., material) it is traveling in. In a vacuum, the electromagnetic radiation travels with the speed of light ($c = 299,792,458\ m/s$, often rounded to $3 \cdot 10^8\ m/s$ or $3 \cdot 10^5 km/s$). The refractive index n of a material is defined as the ratio of the speed of light in vacuum c and the speed of light (velocity) in the corresponding medium v (e.g., glass), where $c > v$.

[1] Planck's constant is named after Max Planck (1858–1947). It is a physical constant that relates the energy of a photon with its frequency.

Table 2.1 Important refractive indices

Material	Refractive index n
Vacuum	1
Air	$1.00029 \approx 1$
Water	1.333
CR-39	1.498
Crown glass	1.523
Trivex	1.532
Polycarbonate	1.586
Diamond	2.417

$$n = \frac{c}{v} \tag{2.4}$$

The table above shows refractive indices for air and some common materials used in optometric practice (Table 2.1).

2.2.2 Snell's Law

The change in velocity of light when it travels from e.g. air ($n = 1$) into an optically denser transparent material ($n' > 1$) leads to a deviation from its path.[2] This phenomenon is referred to as refraction. Refraction on plane transparent surfaces occurs when the incidence ray of light enters the medium with an angle of incidence $\theta_1 > 0$. The angle of incidence is the angle between the incident ray on a surface and the line perpendicular to the surface at the

[2]Note that there are various notations for the enumeration/indication of the refractive indices. Some authors use a numbered system to define the refractive indices. For instance, n_1 would refer to the refractive index of the first (primary), n_2 the second (secondary) medium, and so forth. Sometimes it is more intuitive to use a notation where the refractive index of first medium is denoted by n, and the refractive index of the subsequent medium by n'. I will use the latter notation.

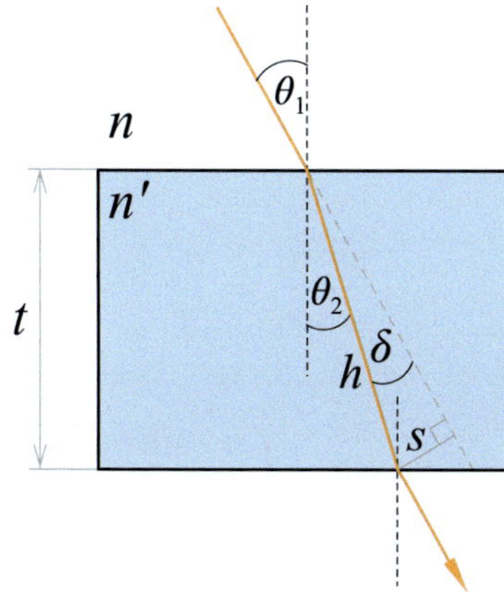

Fig. 2.2 The figure shows the scenrio by which a ray of light (here and throughout illustrated as an orange solid line) in air ($n = 1$) enters a transparent medium (e.g., a block of glass; here and throughout illustrated as the light blue shape) with the refractive index $n' > 1$, and a thickness t. The angles θ_1 and θ_2 denote the angle of incidence and the angle of refraction, respectively. δ is the angle of deviation, h the lenghts of the refracted ray (Note that is also the hypothenus!), and s the lateral displacement. Refraction occurs when $\theta_1 > 0$

point of incidence, i.e., the normal. Here and throughout this book, the normal is represented by a dashed black line (see e.g., Fig. 2.2).

Remember

- If a ray of light travels from an optically less dense into an optically denser transparent material, it is always refracted towards the normal.

Hence, the angle of incidence θ_1 is bigger than the angle of refraction θ_2 ($\theta_1 > \theta_2$).

Snell's law[3] describes the relationship between θ_1 and θ_2.

$$\sin\theta_1 \cdot n = \sin\theta_2 \cdot n' \tag{2.5}$$

∴

$$\frac{\sin\theta_1}{\sin\theta_2} = \frac{n'}{n} \tag{2.6}$$

∴

$$\theta_2 = \sin^{-1}\left(\frac{n \cdot \sin\theta_1}{n'}\right) \tag{2.7}$$

n: Refractive index of primary medium
n': Refractive index of secondary medium
θ_1: Angle of incidence
θ_2: Angle of refraction

2.2.3 Lateral Displacement

The lateral displacement s can be calculated according to:

$$s = \frac{t \cdot \sin(\theta_1 - \theta_2)}{\cos\theta_2} \tag{2.8}$$

2.2.4 Total Internal Reflection

Total internal reflection is a special case of refraction. Light is refracted away from the normal when entering a less dense medium. The critical angle (θ_c) is the angle of incidence at which the angle of refraction equals 90°. Total internal reflection occurs when the angle of incidence exceeds the critical angle (θ_c) as shown in Fig. 2.3.

[3] Named after Willebrord Snellius (1580–1626).

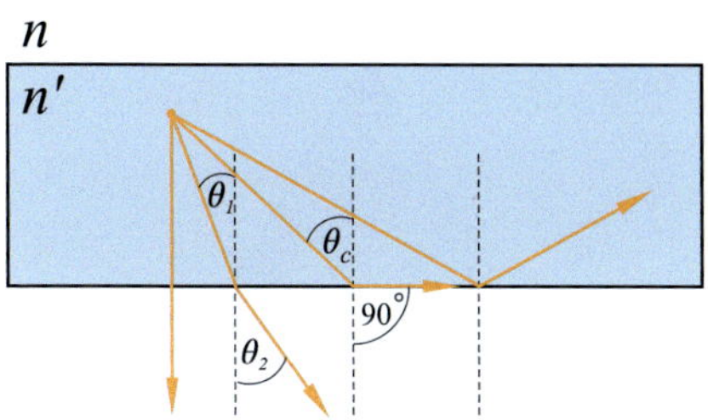

Fig. 2.3 Total internal reflection. Here light travels from the optically denser medium with the refractive index (n') (e.g., glass) into an optically less dense medium with the refractive index n (e.g., air). Note that some textbooks prefer to denote the refractive index of the first material (in this case glass) as n and the refractive index of the second medium (e.g. air) as n'. For the sake of consistency, I continue with the notation employed in Fig. 2.2

The critical angle θ_c can be calculated according to:

$$\sin \theta_c = \frac{n}{n'} \tag{2.9}$$

$\therefore$

$$\theta_c = \sin^{-1} \frac{n}{n'} \tag{2.10}$$

2.2.5 Refraction by Prisms

Transparent optical elements with flat polished surfaces, where at least two surfaces are not parallel are called prisms. Prisms play an imporant role in physical and visual optics and have many applications in optometric and ophthalmic practice (e.g., the correction of diplopia and fusion problems, see Sect. 4.5 and Chap. 9), and in optical instruments

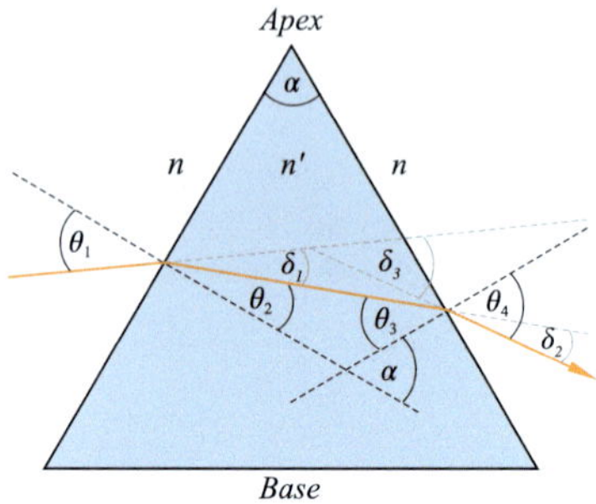

Fig. 2.4 The figure shows a schematic of a ray of light refracted by a triangular prism with an apical angle α. θ_1 denotes the angle of incidence on the first surface, θ_2 the angle of refraction on the first surface, δ_1 the angle of deviation at the first surface, θ_3 the angle of incidence on the second surface, θ_4 is the angle of refraction on the second surface, δ_2 the angle of deviation on the second surface, and δ_3 is the angle of overall deviation

(e.g., Porro prisms[4]). Figure 2.4 shows an illustration of a triangular prims.

2.2.5.1 Angle of Deviation

The angle of deviation δ_3 is the angle between the incidence ray and the emergent ray leaving the prism (see Fig. 2.4). δ_3 can be calculated according to the following equations:

$$\delta_3 = \delta_1 + \delta_2 \tag{2.11}$$

$\therefore$

$$\delta_3 = (\theta_1 + \theta_4) - \alpha \tag{2.12}$$

[4]Porro prisms, named after Ignazio Porro (1801–1875), are prisms that utilize total internal reflection (see Sect. 2.2.4) to alter the orienation of an image (e.g., inversion). Porro prisms are traditionally used in binoculars.

2.2.5.2 Minimum Angle of Deviation

The minimum angle of deviation occurs when the angle of incidence at the first surface θ_1 is equal to the angle of refraction at the second surface θ_4 ($\theta_1 = \theta_4$).

$$\delta_{min} = 2 \cdot \sin^{-1}\left(n' \cdot \left(\frac{\alpha}{2}\right)\right) - \alpha \tag{2.13}$$

The minimum angle of deviation (δ_{min}) can be used to calculate the refractive index of the prism (here n').

$$n' = \frac{\sin(\frac{\alpha+\delta_{min}}{2})}{\sin(\frac{\alpha}{2})} \tag{2.14}$$

2.2.6 Refraction on Curved (Spherical) Surfaces

So far, we have established that refraction occurs when a ray of light enters a transparent medium with an angle of incidence $\theta_1 > 0$, but we conly considered flat surfaces. However, in optics and optometric practice, we often deal with optical surfaces that are curved. For simplicity we consider the curved surfaces to be spherical, i.e., the radii around the center have the same length. The radius of a circle or sphere is any line that connects the center C with the perimeter.[5] A spherical curved surface has an infinite number of radii with equal length along its perimenter (arc length), and the normal can be considered as an extension of the radius.

[5] Note, however, that ophthalmic lenses and lenses in optical instruments are often aspherical, i.e., the radii vary. The advantage of aspherical optical surfaces is that they can reduce optical aberrations (see Sect. 4.2.4).

2.2.6.1 Sign Convention

A curved optical surface can be convex or concave. Figure 2.5 shows the sign convention for radii on a convex (left) and concave (right) surface.

Remember
- The radius r of a convex surface is always positive, whereas the radius of a concave surfaces is always negative.

2.2.6.2 Calculating the Power at Curved Surfaces

Every curved optical surface has a refractive power F that is dependent on the curvature of the surface and the refractive index n' of the material and the surrounding medium n. For spherical surfaces the curvature κ is simply the inverse or reciprocal of the radius r.

$$\kappa = \frac{1}{r} \tag{2.15}$$

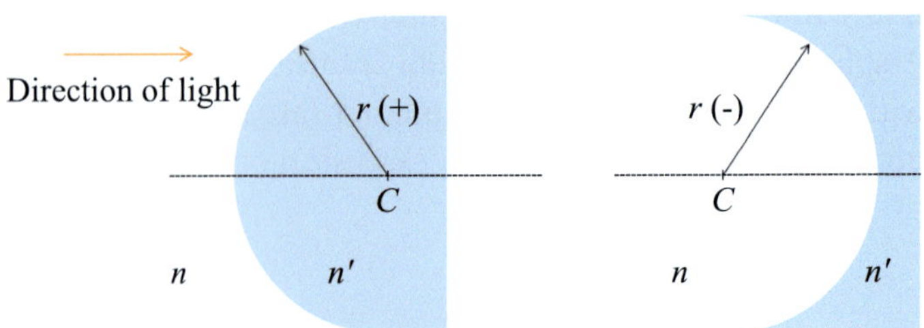

Fig. 2.5 Refraction: Sign convention

The refractive power F of the surface can be calculated according to:

$$F = \frac{n' - n}{r} \tag{2.16}$$

F: Refractive power
r: Radius $[m]$
n: Refractive index of surrounding medium
n': Refractive index of material

Remember

- The radius r is always measured in metres $[m]$.
- Hence, the unit of the refractive[a] power is $^1/_m$, which in optics is referred to as diopter D.

[a]And reflective power, see Sect. 2.3.

Figure 2.6 shows ray diagrams for a convex (left) and a concave lens (right). Convex lenses are often illustrated by a vertical line with arrowheads pointing outwards, whereas concave lenses are represented as a vertical line with arrowheads pointing inwards. For each lens we can define a first principal focus F (primary focal point) and a second principal focus F' (secondary focal point). For thin lenses, where we ignore the width of the lens for the sake of simplicity, the distance between the lens and the first principal focus F is the first focal length f, and the distance between the lens and the second principal focus F' is the second focal length f'. Note that the locations of first and second principal foci are on opposing sides for convex and concave lenses.

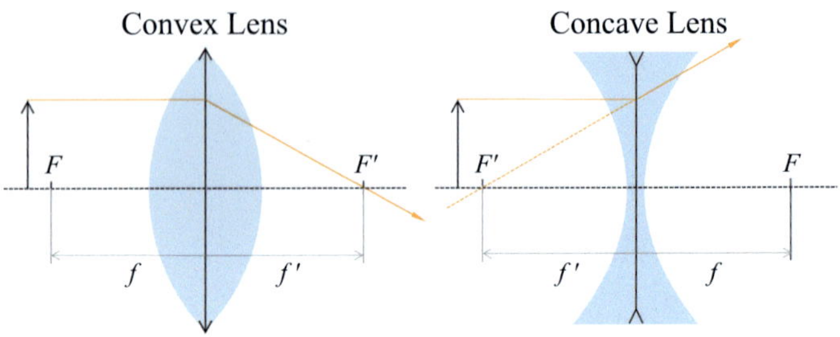

Fig. 2.6 Image formation–lenses

F: First principal focus (not to be mistaken with the refractive power)
F': Second principal focus
f: First focal length/object focal length
f': Second focal length/image focal length

Remember

- The convention is that light always travels from the left to the right.
- Convex lenses are converging lenses.
- Concave lenses are diverging lenses.

2.2.6.3 Image Formation–Lenses

The position and properties of an image created by a lens or lens system are dependent on the refractive power of the lens and, therefore, its focal length as well as its distance from the lens. Figure 2.7 shows three ray diagrams of how to construct the image for convex lenses, and Fig. 2.8 for concave lenses. The object is illustrated as the upright arrow. l denotes the distance of the object from the lens and l' the distance of the image from the lens.

The position of the image can be constructed by utilizing a combination of three different types of rays.

1. Principal ray
2. F ray
3. F' ray

Any two of the three types of rays can be used to construct the image.

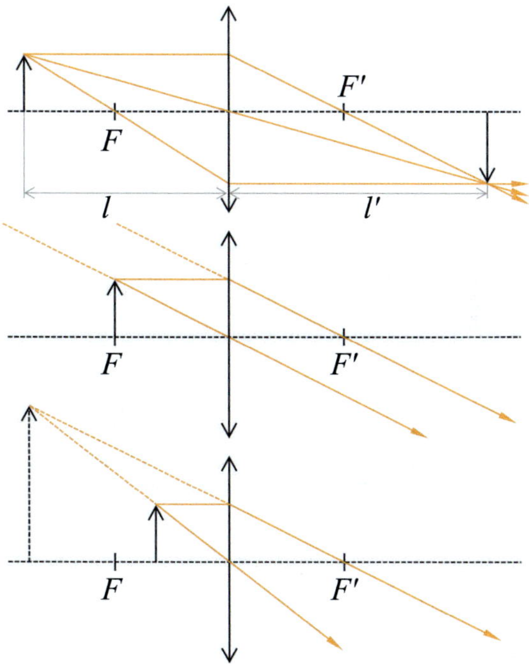

Fig. 2.7 Top diagram: $l > f$–The image is real and inverted. Middle diagram: $l = f$–The image is at infinity, i.e., the emerging rays are parallel. Bottom diagram: $l < f$–The image is upright and virtual

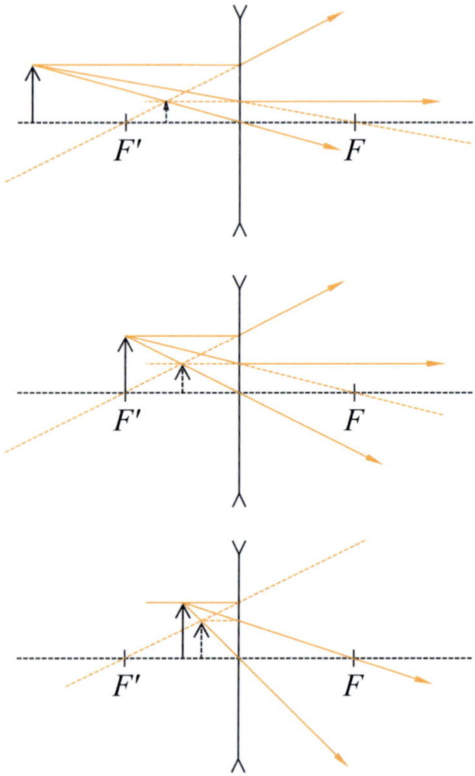

Fig. 2.8 Top diagram: $l > f$–The image is virtual, upright and smaller than the object. Middle diagram: $l = f$–The image is virtual, upright and smaller than the object. Bottom diagram: $l < f$–The image is virtual, upright and smaller than the object

Remember

- All rays are drawn from the tip of the object to the tip of the image.
- The principal ray passes undeviated through the center of the lens (nodal point).
- The *F* ray passes through the first principal focus *F* and emerges from the lens as a ray parallel to the optic axis (paraxial).

- The F' ray is parallel to the optic axis and emerges from the lens as a ray that passes through the second principal focus F' .

Images can be real or virtual. Real images are formed when the emerging rays converge. Real images can be projected onto a screen. Virtual images, on the other hand, are images that are formed when the emerging rays diverge. The virtual image is formed at the point of apparent convergence. The rays converging to a virtual image, and virtual images themselves, are usally drawn as dotted or dashed lines (dashed here). Virtual images can not be formed onto a screen, because divergent rays never converge.

Table 2.2 shows a complete summary of image characteristics.

Table 2.2 Image characteristics–lenses

Type of lens	Object position	Image position	Nature of image	Size of image
Converging	$< f$	Same side of lens	Virtual, upright	Larger
Converging	At F	At ∞		
Converging	Between f & $2f$	Between $2f'$ & ∞	Real, inverted	Larger
Converging	At $2f$	At $2f'$	Real, inverted	Same
Converging	Between $2f$ & ∞	Between f' & $2f'$	Real, inverted	Smaller
Converging	At ∞	At F'	Real, inverted	
Diverging	$< \infty$	$< f'$	Virtual, upright	Smaller
Diverging	At ∞	At F'	Virtual	

2.2.7 Thin Lens Equations

Figure 2.9 shows a ray diagram of a thin lens with an object with a height h at a distance $x + f$, which produces an image with a height h' at a distance $x' + f'$.

We can therefore derive the following relationships:

$$x \cdot x' = f \cdot f' \tag{2.17}$$

$\therefore$

$$\frac{f}{x} = -\frac{x'}{f'} \tag{2.18}$$

We can also derive an equation to relate the object height h, image height h' with x and f'.

$$\frac{h}{h'} = -\frac{x'}{f'} \tag{2.19}$$

The above-mentioned relationship can also be expressed as the **lens formula**,

$$\frac{1}{f} = \frac{1}{u} + \frac{1}{v} \tag{2.20}$$

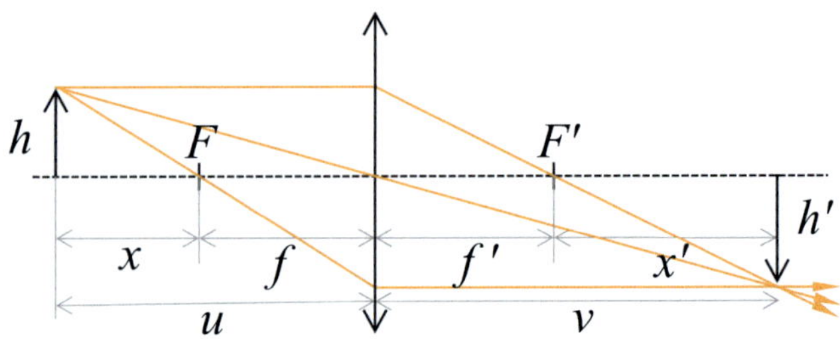

Fig. 2.9 Relationship between focal length f, object distance u, and image distance v

where u denotes the distance of the object to the optical center of the lens (object distance), v the distance of the image to the optical center of the lens (image distance), and f is the distance measured from the principal focus from the optical center of the lens (focal length).

2.2.7.1 Step-Along Method

The position of an image and the refractive power of the lens F can also be calculated using the step-along method by using the concept of vergence. The vergence is the curvature of the wavefront. One can distinguish between the vergence in L (incident vergence) and the vergence out L' (exit vergence). The vergence is dependent on the refractive index n or n' of the medium and the distance from the object to the optical surface l, or the distance between the image and the lens l'. The vergence in and out are illustrated by the yellow arcs symbolising the curvature of the wavefront in Fig. 2.10.

$$L = \frac{n}{l} \tag{2.21}$$

$$L' = \frac{n'}{l'} \tag{2.22}$$

$$\frac{1}{l'} = \frac{1}{l} + \frac{1}{f} \tag{2.23}$$

$\therefore$

$$L' = L + F \tag{2.24}$$

Hence, the refractive power F of the lens can be calculated according to:

$$F = L' - L \tag{2.25}$$

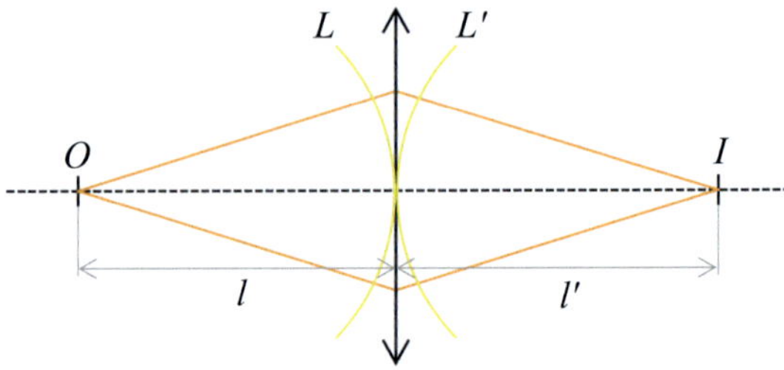

Fig. 2.10 The figure shows the vergence in L and vergence out L' illustrated as the yellow arcs

L: Vergence in (incident vergence) $[D]$
L': Vergence out (exit vergence) $[D]$
l: Distance to object $[m]$
l': Distance to image $[m]$
F: Refractive Power $[D]$
n: Refractive index medium
n': Refractive index surrounding medium

The step-along method can also be applied to calculate the position of an image for a lens system (l'_2 in Fig. 2.12). It is absolutely crucial to adhere to the sign convention, which is summarized in Fig. 2.11.

Remember

- The object is typically located in front of the first lens.
- Note that under these circumstances the distance to the object l [m] is negative.

$$L = \frac{n}{l} \tag{2.26}$$

$$L' = \frac{n'}{l'} \tag{2.27}$$

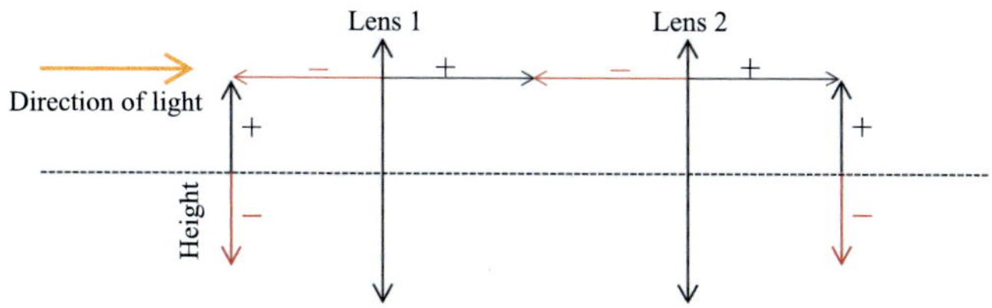

Fig. 2.11 Sign convention

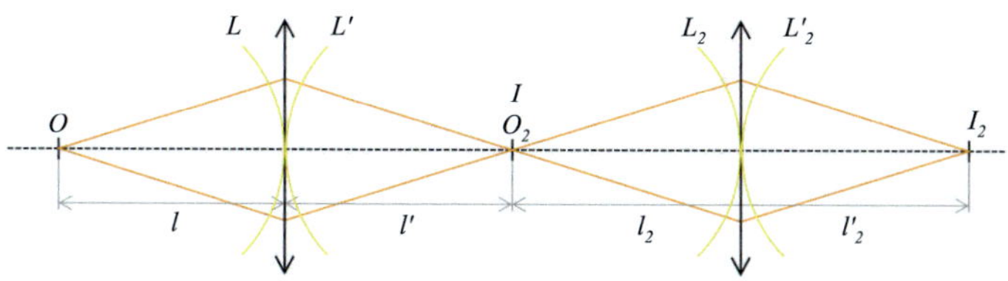

Fig. 2.12 Nomenclature for the step-along method for two lenses

$$l_2 = l' - d \tag{2.28}$$

where d is the distance between the two lenses [m].

$$L_2 = \frac{n'}{l_2} \tag{2.29}$$

where n' is the refractive index of the surrounding medium.[6]

$$L_2' = F_2 + L_2 \tag{2.30}$$

where F_2 is the refractive power of the second lens.

$$l_2' = \frac{n'}{L_2'} \tag{2.31}$$

[6]The refractive index can be different from air.

2.2.8 The Power of a Lens System

For a thin lens system the total power of the lens system is often defined as the exit vergence of light when the incident vergence is zero (parallel light). This is referred to as the back vertex power (F_v').

2.2.8.1 Back Vertex Power Equation

The back vertex power F_v' for thin lenses can be calculated according the following equation.

$$F_v' = \frac{F_1 + F_2 - d \cdot F_1 \cdot F_2}{1 - d \cdot F_1} \tag{2.32}$$

F_v': Back vertex power $[D]$
F_1: Power of the first lens $[D]$
F_2: Power of the second lens $[D]$
d: Distance between the two lenses $[m]$

2.2.8.2 Front Vertex Power

The front vertex power (F_v) is the emergent vergence to the lens system when the exit vergence is zero (parallel light).

$$F_v = \frac{F_1 + F_2 - d \cdot F_1 \cdot F_2}{1 - d \cdot F_2} \tag{2.33}$$

F_v: Front vertex power $[D]$

2.2.8.3 Back Vertex Distance

The back vertex distance refers to the distance between the back vertex of the spectacle lens (or contact lens) and the corneal apex. In the case of a contact lens the back vertex distance would be zero. Changes in the back vertex distance require a change in F'_v, and can be calculated according to the following equations.

$$F'_{v2} = \frac{F'_{v1}}{1 + (d_2 - d_1 \cdot F'_{v1})} \tag{2.34}$$

$$\Delta d = d_2 - d_1 \tag{2.35}$$

$$F'_{v2} = \frac{F'_{v1}}{1 + (\Delta d \cdot F'_{v1})} \tag{2.36}$$

F'_{v1}: old back vertex power $[D]$
F'_{v2}: new back vertex power $[D]$
d_1: old back vertex distance $[m]$
d_2: new back vertex distance $[m]$

2.2.9 Thick Lenses

When the thickness or width of a lens is no longer regarded as negligible, then the lens is considered thick. Even contact lenses can be considered thick lenses. The properties of a thick lens is dependent on the surface curvatures, the refractive index n of the lens material (and the surrounding medium), and the thickness t of the lens.

For a thick lens we also use the back vertex power F'_v (Fig. 2.13).

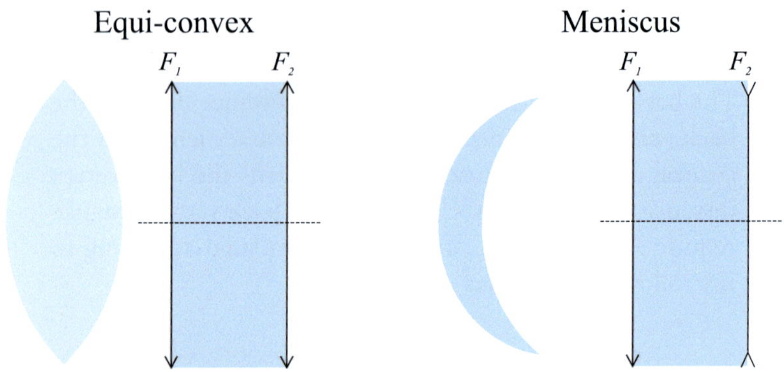

Fig. 2.13 The figure shows a equi-convex lens (left) composed of two positive surfaces and and a meniscus lens, which is composed of a positive front surface F_1 and a negative back surface F_2

The back vertex power (and front vertex power) of the lens is dependent on:

- the front surface power F_1
- the back surface power F_2
- the lens thickness t
- the refractive index of the medium n

2.2.10 The Power of Thick Lens

2.2.10.1 Back Vertex Power

$$F_v' = \frac{F_1 + F_2 - (t/n') \cdot F_1 \cdot F_2}{1 - (t/n') \cdot F_1} \tag{2.37}$$

Below find Eq. 2.37 re-arranged to F_1,F_2, t, n', and the equation for the focal length f'_v.

$$F_1 = \frac{F'_v - F_2}{1 - (t/n') \cdot F_2 + (t/n') \cdot F'_v} \tag{2.38}$$

$$F_2 = \frac{F'_v \cdot (1 - (t/n') \cdot F_1) - F_1}{1 - (t/n') \cdot F_1} \tag{2.39}$$

$$t = \frac{n' \cdot (F_1 + F_2 - F'_v)}{-F_1 \cdot F'_v + F_1 \cdot F_2} \tag{2.40}$$

$$n' = \frac{t \cdot (-F_1 \cdot F'_v + F_1 \cdot F_2)}{(F_1 + F_2 - F'_v)} \tag{2.41}$$

$$f'_v = \frac{n'}{F'_v} \tag{2.42}$$

F'_v: Back vertex power $[D]$
f'_v: Second focal length (distance from back lens to second focal point) $[m]$
F_1: Power of the first lens $[D]$
F_2: Power of the second lens $[D]$
t: Distance between the two surfaces; width of the lens $[m]$
n': Refractive index of lens material

2.2.10.2 Front Vertex Power

$$F_v = \frac{F_1 + F_2 - (t/n') \cdot F_1 \cdot F_2}{1 - (t/n') \cdot F_2} \tag{2.43}$$

$$f_v = -\frac{n}{F_v} \tag{2.44}$$

F_V: Front vertex power $[D]$
f_V: First focal length (distance from front lens to first focal point) $[m]$
n: Refractive index surrounding medium

2.3 Reflection

In optics, the term reflection describes the phenomenon by which a ray of light (or wavefront) changes its direction at the interface of two different media. Depending on the physical properties of the surface of the medium, we can distinguish between diffuse and specular reflection. Here we will mainly focus on specular (mirror-like) reflection, which occurs on polished surfaces, such as mirrors. Total internal reflection is a special type of refraction (see Sect. 2.2.4).

2.3.1 Reflection on Plane Mirrors

Figure 2.14 shows an illustration of a plane mirror. The law of reflection states that the angle of incidence i is equal to the angle of reflection i_r.

Law of reflection

$$i = i_r \tag{2.45}$$

i: Angle of incidence
i_r: Angle of reflection

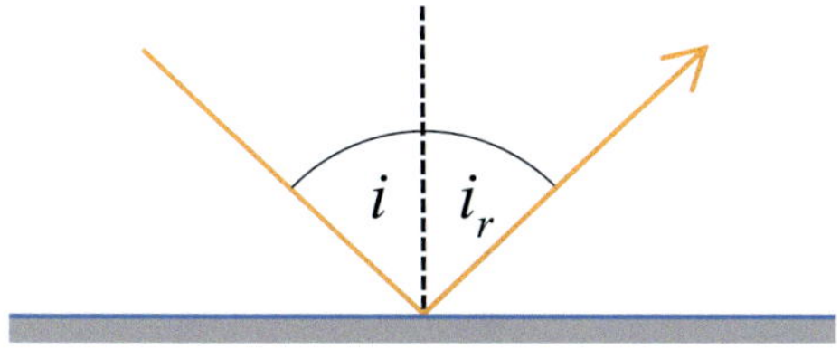

Fig. 2.14 Reflection on plane surfaces

2.3.2 Reflection on Curved (Spherical) Mirrors

Similar to lenses, curved mirrors can be classified as concave and convex mirrors. For simplicity, we only consider spherical mirrors here.[7] Concave mirrors are converging mirrors, whereas convex mirrors are diverging mirrors. Figure 2.15 shows ray diagrams for a concave mirror (left) and a convex mirror (right). For spherical mirrors, the radius r extends from the center of curvature C to the pole (vertex) A. Given the spherical nature of the mirror, it becomes clear that, according to the law of reflection (Eq. 2.45), a paraxial ray will be reflected so that it passes through a point along the optic axis that is located at $^r/_2$. This point is defined as the focal point F of the mirror. The distance between A and F is the focal length f of the mirror.

$$f = \frac{r}{2} \tag{2.46}$$

C: Center of curvature
F: Focal point
A: Pole/Vertex
r: Radius
f: Focal length

[7]Note that similar to ophthalmic lenses, mirrors in optical instruments are often aspherical (e.g., parabolic).

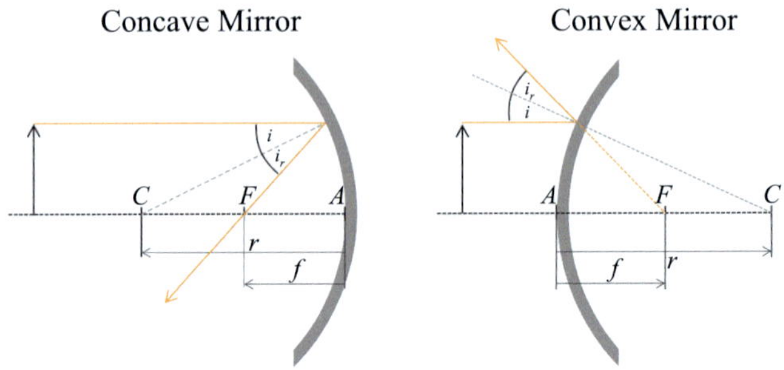

Fig. 2.15 Reflection on curved mirrors

Remember

- Concave mirrors are converging mirrors.
- The radius r of a concave mirror is positive.
- The focal length f of a concave mirror is positive.
- Convex mirrors are diverging mirrors.
- The radius r of a convex mirror is negative.
- The focal length f of a convex mirror is negative.

$$F_r = \frac{1}{f} \tag{2.47}$$

F_r: Reflective power of the mirror

2.3.2.1 Image Formation–Mirrors

Figure 2.16 shows ray diagrams for the image construction for concave mirrors. Mirrors are often illustrated by a vertical line with a semi-circle indicating its curvature (convex or concave). The images in Figs. 2.16 and 2.17 are constructed with the help of three different types of rays.

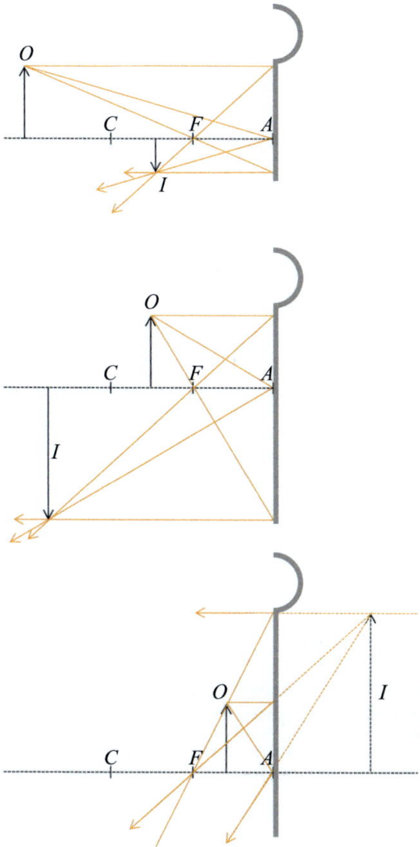

Fig. 2.16 Image formation–concave mirror

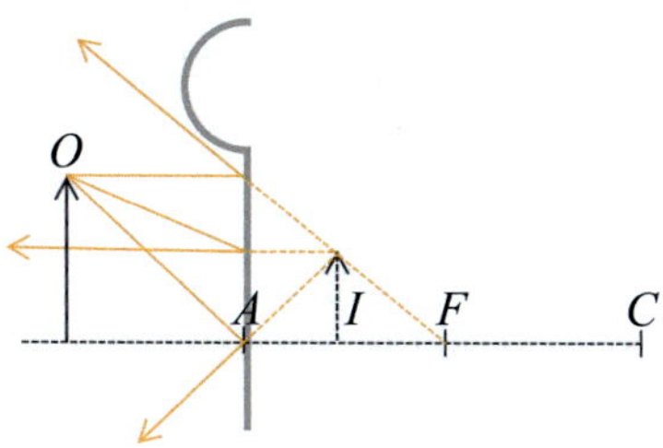

Fig. 2.17 Image formation–convex mirror

Remember

- All rays are drawn from the tip of the object to the tip of the image.
- All rays follow the law of reflection $i = i_r$.
  Hence:
- Rays parallel to the optic axis are reflected through the focal point F.
- Rays passing through the focal point F are reflected parallel to the optic axis.
- Rays passing through the Pole (Vertex) A are reflected in the same angle.
- Rays passing through the center of curvature C will be reflected through C (not shown).

Table 2.3 shows a complete summary of image characteristics for concave and convex mirrors.

Table 2.3 Image characteristics–mirrors

Type of mirror	Object position	Image position	Nature of image	Size of image
Concave	$< f$	Behind the mirror	Virtual, upright	Larger
Concave	At F	At ∞		
Concave	Between C & F	Between C & ∞	Real, inverted	Larger
Concave	At C	At C	Real, inverted	Same
Concave	Between $2f$ & ∞	Between f & $2f$	Real, inverted	Smaller
Concave	At ∞	At F	Real, inverted	
Convex	All positions	Behind the mirror	Virtual upright	Smaller

2.4 Exercises

1. Calculate the wavelength of light traveling with the speed of light (assuming $c = 3 \cdot 10^5 km/s$) and a frequency of 10^{12} *Hz*.
2. A light ray is traveling into a block of Crown Glass ($n = 1.523$) with a width of 4 *cm* surrounded by air. The angle of incidence is 30°. Calculate the angle of refraction.
3. Derive the equation for the lateral deplacement s (see Eq. 2.8 in Sect. 2.2.3).
4. Calculate the angle of deviation when light is incident at 40° on the surface of a block of glass with a refractive index of $n = 1.5$?
5. What is the lateral displacement s if a ray of light hits a block of glass with a refractive index of $n = 1.523$ and a width of $t = 2cm$ with angle of incidence of 30°?
6. An object in air is located $100mm$ away from a surface separating air and glass ($n = 1.5$). The image is formed $10cm$ within the glass. What is the power of the surface?
7. A prism made of glass ($n = 1.523$) and an apical angle of $\alpha = 30°$ is submerged in water ($n = 1.333$). The angle of incidence $\theta = 40°$. Calculate the total angle of deviation?
8. What is the critical angle for total internal reflection to occur within a block of transparent plastic ($n = 1.4$) surrounded by air?
9. A lens system is composed of two lenses, where lens 1 has a refractive power $F_1 = -2D$ and lens 2 a refractive power $F_2 = -1$. The distance between the two lenses is $d = 3cm$. An object is located 25 *cm* in front of lens. Calculate the position of the resulting image with respect to lens 2.
10. A lens system is made up of a $+20.00D$ lens and a $+30.00D$ lens separated by 10 *cm*. The lenses are surrounded by air. Assume a thick lens with a refractive

index $n = 1.523$. What is the back vertex power of the lens system? Find the solution by using both, the step-along method and the formula.

2.5 Further Reading

- Freeman MH, Hull CC. Optics. 11th Edition. Butterworth Heinemann. 2003.
- Lahiri, A. Basic Optics: Principles and Concepts., Elsevier Science. 2016.
- Tunnacliffe AH. Introduction to visual optics. London: Association of british dispensing opticians; 1993.
- Tunnacliffe AH., Hirst, JG, Optics. Association of British Dispensing Opticians. London; 1996.

References

1. Stiles WS, Burch JM. NPL colour-matching investigation: final report (1958). Optica Acta: Int J Optics. 1959;6(1):1–26.
2. Stockman A, Sharpe LT, Fach CC. The spectral sensitivity of the human short-wavelength cones. Vis Res. 1999;39:2901–27.
3. Stockman A, Sharpe LT. The spectral sensitivities of the middle-and long-wavelength-sensitive cones derived from measurements in observers of known genotype. Vis Res. 2000;40(13):1711–37.
4. Brown PK, Wald G. Visual pigments in single rods and cones of the human retina. Science. 1964;144(3614):45–52.

3

Visual Optics

Visual optics will relate the principles of physical optics covered in Chap. 2 to the eye. In the first part of this chapter, I will introduce various common eye models and their properties. This chapter contains many illustrations to visualize the optical properties of ametropias, like myopia, hyperopia, and astigmatism, and associated calculations.

3.1 Schematic Eye Models

A schematic eye model is a paraxial, simplified representation of the optics of the real human eye. It assumes that all of the ocular surfaces are well-centred and that all rays are paraxial. Schematic eye models were derived from actual measurements of eyes. Aberrations that typically occur at all optical surfaces are ignored. In the following, I will summarize the most important schematic eye models and their properties.

G. Schmidtmann, *Clinical Vision Science*,
https://doi.org/10.1007/978-3-031-83321-2_3

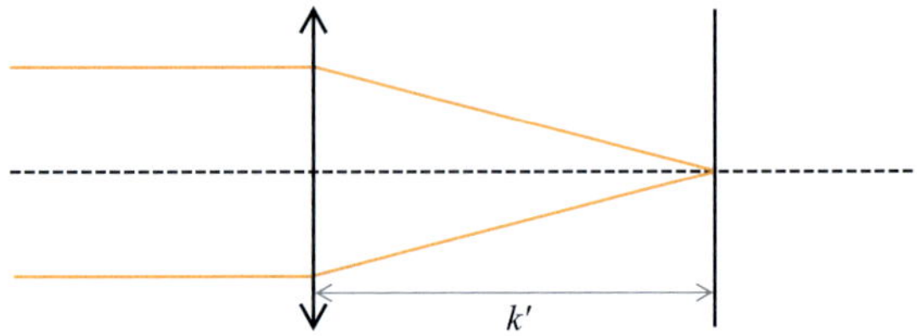

Fig. 3.1 The thin lens eye model consists of a single convex lens with and a screen. The variable k' denotes the axial length

3.1.1 Thin Lens Eye Model

The thin lens eye model is the simplest eye model. It consists of a single thin lens, which represents all the refractive surfaces of the eye and an image screen that represents the retina. A typical dioptric power for the lens representing the non-accommodating emmetropic eye is $+60.00D$. Hence, according to $f' = 1/F$, the axial length k' would be 0.0167 m (Fig. 3.1).

3.1.2 Gullstrand's Reduced Schematic Eye

Gullstrand's[1] reduced schematic eye model assumes only one refracting surface (cornea) (Fig. 3.2). The reduced schematic eye has the same refractive power as the simplified schematic eye model and the exact schematic eye model (see Sects. 3.1.3 and 3.1.4). The dimensions and other characteristics of this eye model are summarized in Table 3.1 [1].

[1] Allvar Gullstrand (1862–1930) was a Swedish ophthalmologist and a professor at the University of Uppsala. He was awarded the Nobel Prize in Physiology or Medicine in 1911.

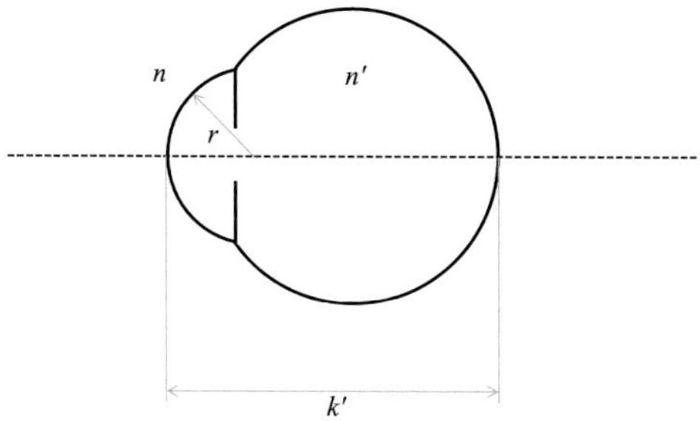

Fig. 3.2 Gullstrand's reduced schematic eye model

Table 3.1 Gullstrand's reduced schematic eye model

Dimensions	[*mm*]
Axial length (k')	22.22
Radii	[*mm*]
cornea (r)	5.56
Refractive index	n
eye (n')	4/3

3.1.3 Gullstrand's Simplified Schematic Eye

Gullstrand's simplified schematic eye assumes three refracting surface (cornea, front & back surface of lens) (Fig. 3.3). The dimensions and other characteristics of this eye model are summarized in Table 3.2 [1].

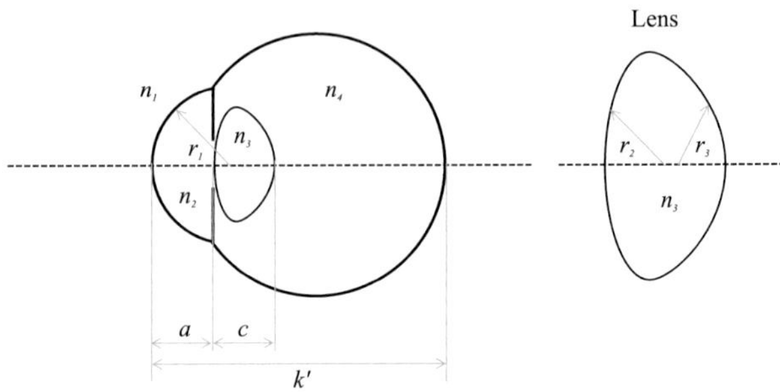

Fig. 3.3 Gullstrand's simplified schematic eye model

Table 3.2 Gullstrand's simplified schematic eye model

Dimensions	*[mm]*
Anterior chamber (a)	3.6
Lens width (c)	3.6
Axial length (k')	24.17
Radii	*[mm]*
Cornea (r_1)	7.8
Anterior lens (r_2)	10.0
Posterior lens (r_3)	–6.0
Cornea (r_4)	7.8
Anterior lens (r_5)	10.0
Posterior lens (r_6)	–6.0
Refractive indices	n
Aqueous humour (n_2)	1.336
Lens (n_3)	1.413
Vitreous (n_4)	1.413

3.1.4 Gullstrand's Exact Schematic Eye

Gullstrand's exact schematic eye is the most complex schematic eye model and assumes six refracting surface (Fig. 3.4). The dimensions and other characteristics of this eye model are summarized in Table 3.3 [1].

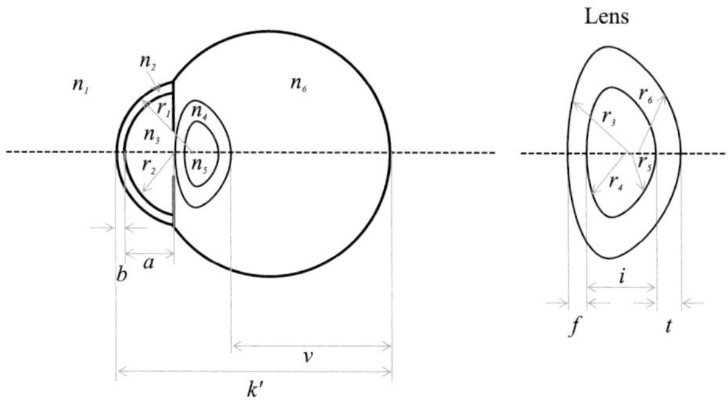

Fig. 3.4 Gullstrand's exact schematic eye model

Table 3.3 Gullstrand's exact schematic eye model

Dimensions	[*mm*]
Width of cornea (b)	0.5
Anterior chamber (a)	3.1
Lens cortex anterior (f)	0.546
Lens nucleus (i)	2.419
Lens cortex posterior (t)	0.635
Vitreous (v)	17.185
Axial length (k')	24.385
Radii	[*mm*]
Cornea anterior (r_1)	7.7
Cornea posterior (r_2)	6.8
Lens cortex anterior (r_3)	10.0
Lens nucleus anterior (r_4)	7.911
Lens nucleus posterior (r_5)	–5,76
Lens cortex posterior (r_6)	–6.0
Refractive Indices	n
Cornea (n_2)	1.376
Aqueous humour (n_3)	1.336
Lens cortex (n_4)	1.386
Lens nucleus (n_5)	1.406
Vitreous (n_6)	1.336

3.2 Emmetropia

The term emmetropia describes the refractive state of the eye in which parallel rays of light entering the eye are focused on the retina and create a focused image on the retina. A more formal defintion is shown in the box below. Emmetropia is illustrated in Fig. 3.5.

Remember

An unaccommodated eye is emmetropic if:

- the second focal point f_e' conincides with the centre of the fovea M'
- if the far point M_r is at infinity (∞)
- the axial lenght k' is equal to the focal length f_e'
- Hence, the second prinipal focus F_e' coincides with the fovea M'

Equations 3.1 and 3.2 can be used to convert from a specular refraction F_{sp} to an ocular refraction K.

$$F_{sp} = \frac{K}{1 + (d \cdot K)} \tag{3.1}$$

$$K = \frac{F_{sp}}{1 + (d \cdot F_{sp})} \tag{3.2}$$

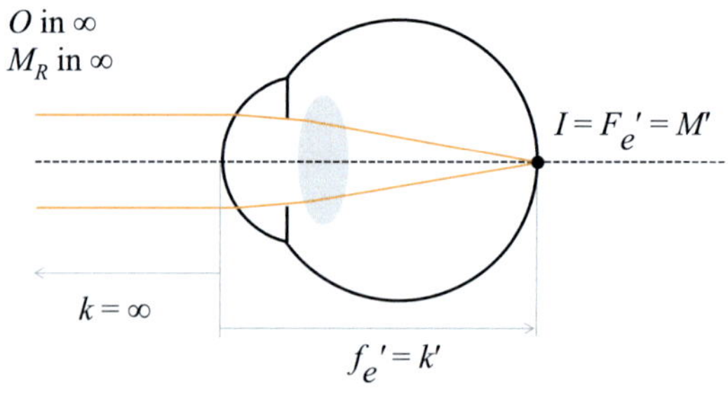

Fig. 3.5 Emmetropia

O: Object

I: Image

M_R: Far point

k: Far point distance

M': Fovea

F'_e: Second principal focus (e refers to eye)

f'_e: Focal length

k': Axial length

K: Ocular refraction

F_{sp}: Specular refraction

3.3 Changes in Back Vertex Distance

It is important to measure the back vertex distance d. Changes in back vertex distance d result in changes in back vertex power F'_v. These changes are dependent on the back vertex power F'_v and the back vertex distance. In general, the higher F'_v, the higher are the required changes. These changes can be significant, as illustrated in Table 3.4. The following equations can be used to calculate the required changes.

$$F'_{v2} = \frac{F'_{v1}}{1 + (d_2 - d_1) \cdot F'_{v1}} \tag{3.3}$$

$$F'_{v2} = \frac{F'_{v1}}{1 + \Delta d \cdot F'_{v1}} \tag{3.4}$$

Alternatively, one could also use the following equation to calculate the back vertex power required for a contact lens F'_{cl} for a given back vertex power for glasses spectacles F'_{sp}.

Table 3.4 Changes in back vertex power in D between spectacles $d = 10$ *mm* and contact lenses $d = 0$ *mm*

F'_{sp}	F'_{cl}	F'_{sp}	F'_{cl}
5.00	5.26	–5.00	–4.76
5.25	5.54	–5.25	–4.99
5.50	5.82	–5.50	–5.21
5.75	6.10	–5.75	–5.44
6.00	6.38	–6.00	–5.66
6.25	6.67	–6.25	–5.88
6.50	6.95	–6.50	–6.10
6.75	7.24	–6.75	–6.32
7.00	7.53	–7.00	–6.54
7.25	7.82	–7.25	–6.76
7.50	8.11	–7.50	–6.98
7.75	8.40	–7.75	–7.19
8.00	8.70	–8.00	–7.41
8.25	8.99	–8.25	–7.62
8.50	9.29	–8.50	–7.83
8.75	9.59	–8.75	–8.05
9.00	9.89	–9.00	–8.26
9.25	10.19	–9.25	–8.47
9.50	10.50	–9.50	–8.68
9.75	10.80	–9.75	–8.88
10.00	11.11	–10.00	–9.09

$$F'_{cl} = \frac{F'_{sp}}{1 - d \cdot F'_{sp}} \tag{3.5}$$

F'_{v1}: Back vertex power 1

F'_{v2}: Back vertex power 2

F'_{cl}: Back vertex power contact lens

F'_{sp}: Back vertex power spectacles

d: Back vertex distance

3.4 Ametropia

An eye is ametrope when the far point M_R is not at infinity. An object located at infinity (∞) does not create a point-like (focused) image on the retina. The following sections will summarize the most important ametropias (myopia, hyperopia, and astigmatism). Ametropias are characeterized by an imbalance of refractive power of the eye and the length of the eye.

3.5 Myopia

Myopia, also commonly called short or near-sightedness, is a condition where the far point M_R is located at a finite distance in front of the eye ($m_R < 0$). In myopia the eye is too long or the refractive power is too high. Consequently, a point at infinity will be in focus in front of the retina. Myopia is illustrated in Fig. 3.6.

Remember

An unaccommodated eye is myopic if:

- the second focal point f_e' is in front of centre of the fovea M' ($k' > f_e'$)
- the far point M_r is at a finite distance in front of the eye ($m_R < 0$)
- Myopia is corrected with negative (diverging) specatacle lenses

$$k = f'_{sp} - d \tag{3.6}$$

$$K = \frac{1}{k} \tag{3.7}$$

$$f'_{sp} = k + d \tag{3.8}$$

$$F'_{sp} = \frac{1}{f'_{sp}} \tag{3.9}$$

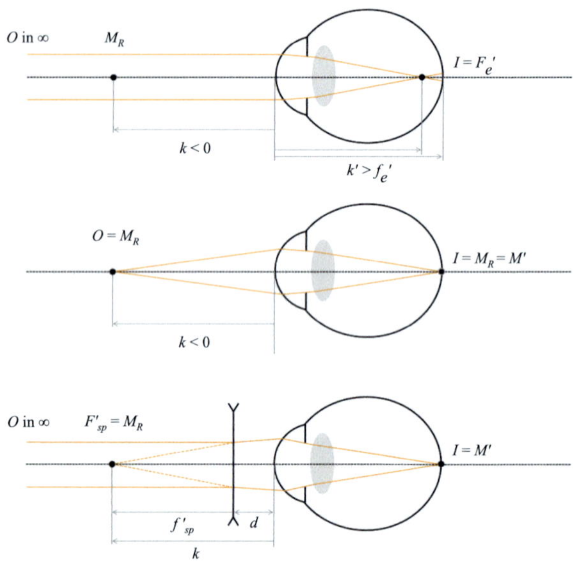

Fig. 3.6 The figure shows an illustration of a myopic eye and its correction

O: Object

I: Image

M_R: Far point

k: Far point distance

M': Fovea

F'_e: Second principal focus (e refers to eye)

f'_e: Focal length (eye)

F'_{sp}: Second principal focus (sp refers to lens / spectacles)

f'_{sp}: Focal length of lens

K: Ocular refraction

d: Back vertex distance

3.6 Hyperopia/Hypermetropia

Hyperopia, also hypermetropia or far-sightedness, is a type of ametropia where the far point M_R is located at a finite distance behind the eye ($m_R > 0$). In hyperopia, the refractive power of the eye is too weak, or the length of the eye is too short. Hyperopia and its correction are illustrated in Fig. 3.7.

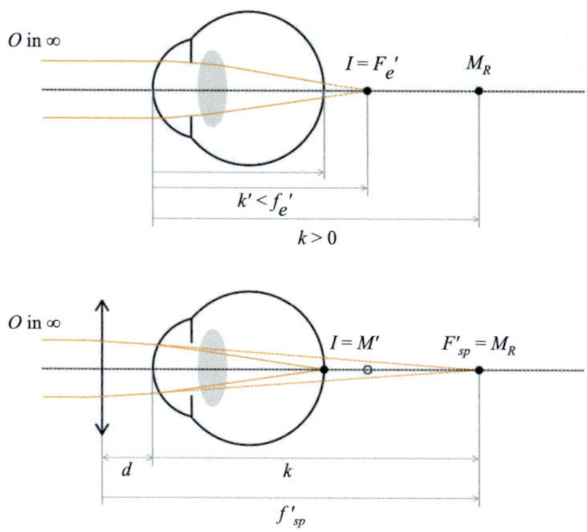

Fig. 3.7 Hyperopia

O: Object

I: Image

M_R: Far point

k: Far point distance

M': Fovea

F'_e: Second principal focus (e refers to eye)

f'_e: Focal length (eye)

F'_{sp}: Second principal focus (sp refers to lens / spectacles)

f'_{sp}: Focal length of lens

K: Ocular refraction

d: Back vertex distance

Remember

An unaccommodated eye is hyperopic if:

- the second focal point f'_e is behind the centre of the fovea M' ($k' < f'_e$)
- the far point M_R is at a finite distance behind the eye ($m_R > 0$)
- Hyperopia is corrected with positive (converging) specatacle lenses

$$k = f'_{sp} - d \tag{3.10}$$

$$K = \frac{n}{k} \tag{3.11}$$

$$f'_{sp} = k + d \tag{3.12}$$

$$F'_{sp} = \frac{n}{f'_{sp}} \tag{3.13}$$

3.7 Astigmatism

In the case of astigmatism, the radii of the cornea are not uniform; the cornea is aspherical.[2] Hence, the refractive power of the cornea is different in different meridians. This results in an optical system that produces focal lines, instead of a single focal point or focus. Astigmatisms can be classified as regular or irregular. In the case of regular astigmatism, the focal lines are perpendicular to each other (90° apart). The irregular shape of the cornea in the case of, e.g. a keratoconus or corneal scaring, can result in a scenario where the focal lines are not perpendicular to each other. This is referred to as an irregular astigmatism. In this chapter, I will only discuss regular astigmatisms. Figure 3.8 shows an illustration of astigmatism.

Astigmatism results in a blur ellipse rather than a blur circle. The point halfway between the two focal lines is referred to as the circle of least confusion. The magnitude of astigmatism is defined as the difference between the maximum and minimum meridial powers and is referred to as the cylinder. We can distinguish between five different types of regular astigmatisms, depending on the locations of the focal lines with repect to the retina. These are illustrated in Fig. 3.9.

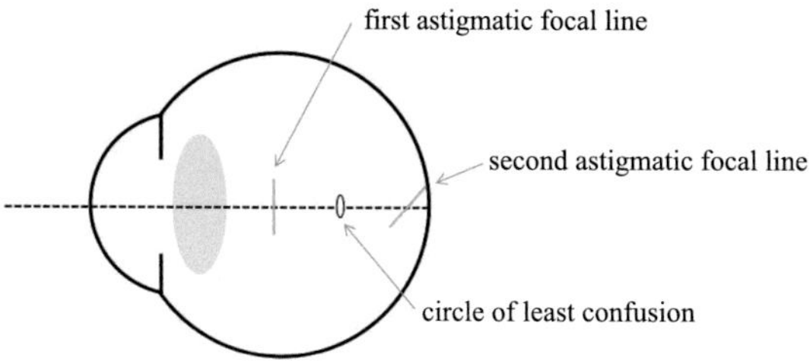

Fig. 3.8 Astigmatism

[2]Here we assume that it is the cornea that produces an astigmatism. However, the crystalline lens can also contribute.

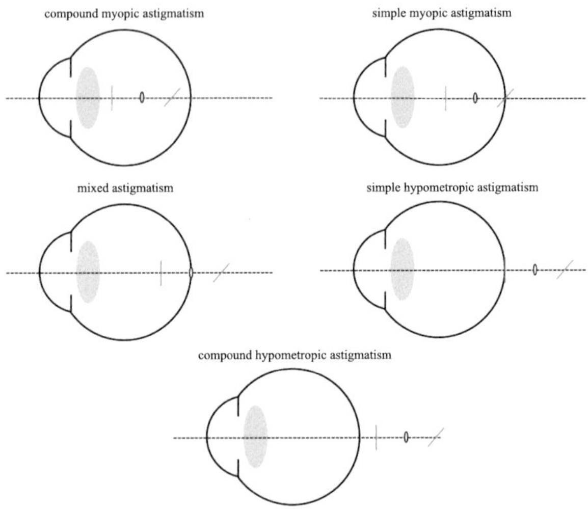

Fig. 3.9 Types of astigmatism

Remember

The types of regular astigmatism are:

- Compound myopic astigmatism: Both focal lines are located in front of the retina (-1.50 DS/-1.50DC x 90)
- Simple myopic astigmatism: One focal line is located in front of the retina, the other one is directly on the retina (plano/-1.50DC x 90)
- Mixed astigmatism: One focal line is located in front of the retina, the other behind the retina (-1.50DS/+3.00 x 90)[a]
- Simple hypermetropic astigmatism: One focal line is located is directly on the retina, the other one behind the retina (plano/+1.50DC x 90)

- Compound hypermetropic astigmatism: Both focal lines are located behind front of the retina (+1.50 DS/+1.50DC x 90)

[a]The circle of least confusion can be located on the retina, but does not have to be located there.

3.8 Accommodation

Accommodation is the ability of the eye to change its refractive power to focus on objects at various distances. Positive accommodation refers to an increase in refractive power, whereas negative accommodation refers to a decrease in the eye's refractive power. The overall amount of possible accommodation, i.e. change in refractive power, is called amplitude of accommodation. Figure 3.10 shows important points and distances of accommodation.

Remember

Classification of Accommodation

- **Tonic accommodation**: The amount of accommodation in a resting state, without stimulus.
- **Convergence accommodation**: The amout of accommodation resulting from convergence.
- **Proximal accommodation**: The amount of accommodation triggered by the awarness of the proximity of an object in the near.
- **Reflex accommodation**: Involuntary accommodation as a results of a blurry retinal image.
- **Voluntary accommodation**: Voluntary accommodation, independent of a stimulus.

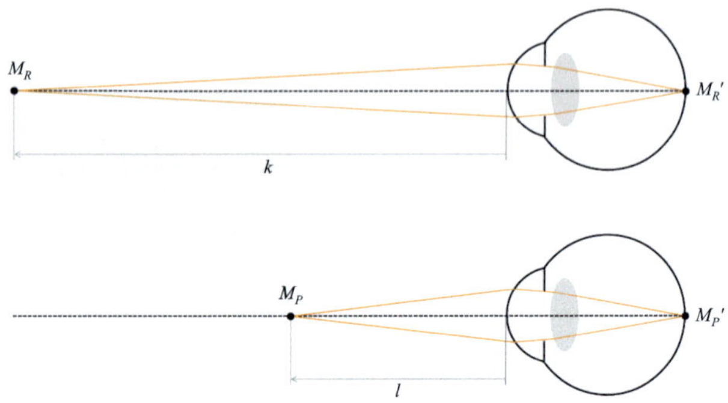

Fig. 3.10 The figure shows the true far point M_R, the true near point M_P and the range of accommodation as the grey-shaded area

K: Ocular refraction

k: Far point distance

F_{sp}: Specular refraction

d: Back vertex distance

l: True near point distance

Remember

Accommodation–Spectacles vs. Contact Lenses

- A myope wearing contact lenses will have to accommodate more than if corrected with spectacles.
- A hyperope wearing contact lenses will have to accommodate less than if corrected with spectacles.

3.8.1 Accommodation Curves

Presbyopia describes the decrease in the amplitude of accommodation with age. Figure 3.11 shows the mean, maximum and minimum amplitude of accommodation as a function of age [1,2]. Table 3.5 shows the maximum, minimum and

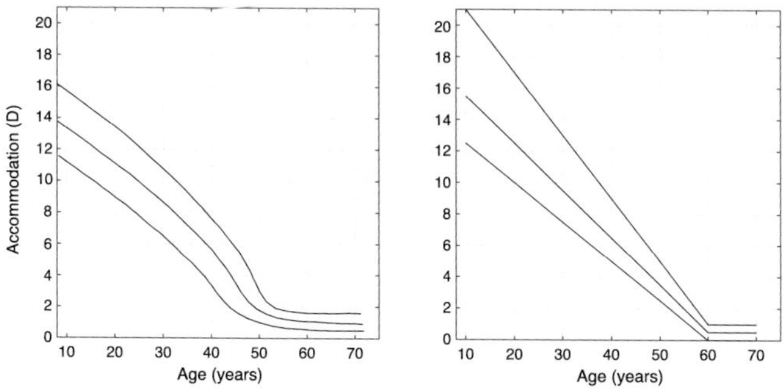

Fig. 3.11 The figure shows the curves describing the mean (A_{mean}), maximim (A_{max}) and minimum (A_{min}) according to Duane (left) [2] and Hoffstetter (right) [3]

mean monocular amplitude of accommodation as a function of age. These can be estimated by the Eqs. 3.14–3.16 below.

$$A_{min} = 15 - (0.25 \cdot age) \tag{3.14}$$

$$A_{mean} = 18.5 - (0.30 \cdot age) \tag{3.15}$$

$$A_{max} = 25.0 - (0.40 \cdot age) \tag{3.16}$$

A_{min}: Minimum amplitude of accommodation

A_{mean}: Mean amplitude of accommodation

A_{max}: Maximum amplitude of accommodation

Table 3.5 Monocular amplitude of accommodation

Age [years]	A_{min} [D]	A_{mean} [D]	A_{max} [D]
10	12.50	15.50	21.00
20	10.00	12.50	17.00
30	7.50	9.50	13.00
40	5.00	6.50	9.00
45	3.75	5.00	7.00
50	2.50	3.50	5.00
55	1.25	2.00	3.00
60	0.00	0.50	1.00

3.9 Exercises

1. Calculate the change in back vertex power required for specular refraction of $-7D$ when the back vertex distance is changed from 15 mm to 5 mm.
2. A myopic patient with a prescription of $-5.00D$ is corrected for the distance with a spectacle lens placed at 10 mm in front of the eye. Calculate the accommodation (A) required when viewing an object at 30 cm in front of the spectacle lens. If this eye was then corrected with a contact lens, how much accommodation is required when viewing the same object?

3.10 Further Reading

- Bennett AG, Rabbetts RB. Bennett and Rabbetts' clinical visual optics. Elsevier Health Sciences; 1998.
- Freeman MH, Hull CC. Optics. 11th Edition. Butterworth Heinemann. 2003.
- Keirl A, Christie C, editors. Clinical optics and refraction: A guide for optometrists, contact lens opticians and

dispensing opticians. Butterworth Heinemann, Elsevier Health Sciences; 2007.
- Tunnacliffe AH. Introduction to visual optics. London: Association of british dispensing opticians; 1993.

References

1. Brodie, S.E. 2022–2023 Basic and Clinical Science Course, Section 03: Clinical Optics and Vision, Rehabilitation Print; American Academy of Ophthalmology: San Francisco, CA, USA, 2022; ISBN 9781681045436.
2. Duane A. Studies in monocular and binocular accommodation with their clinical applications. Am J Ophthalmol. 1922;5(11):865–77.
3. Hofstetter HW. A comparison of Duane's and Donder's tables of the amplitude of accommodation. Optomet Vis Sci. 1944;21(9):345–863.

4

Ophthalmic Lenses

In the following chapter, I will summarize some useful information about the types and properties of ophthalmic lenses. Furthermore, I will introduce the concept of spherocylindrical and prismatic lenses.

4.1 Types of Lenses

Positive (plus, converging) ophthalmic lenses are thickest at the lens center and thinnest at the lens edge. These lenses are used to correct hyperopia (hypermetropia, far-sightedness) and presbyopia (see Sects. 3.6 and 3.8). Conversely, negative (minus, diverging) lenses are thinnest at the lens center and thickest towards the edge of the lens. These types of lenses are used to correct myopia (short-sightedness; see Sect. 3.5).

Figure 4.1 shows some common ophthalmic lens shapes and their terminology.

G. Schmidtmann, *Clinical Vision Science*,
https://doi.org/10.1007/978-3-031-83321-2_4

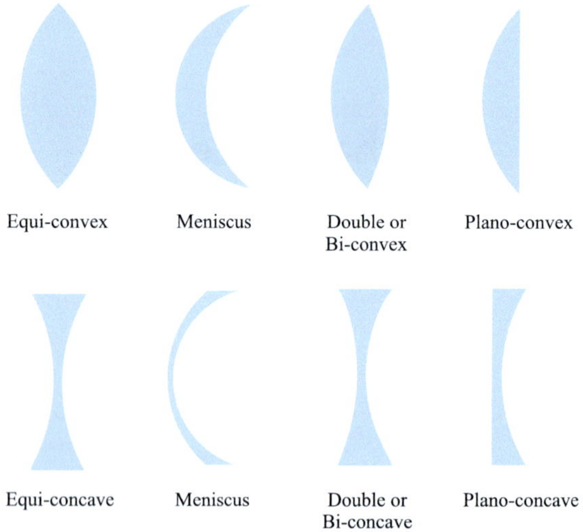

Fig. 4.1 The figure shows various types of common ophthalmic lenses and the corresponding terminology. Convex (converging) lenses are shown in the top panel and concave (diverging) lenses are shown in the bottom panel

4.2 Ophthalmic Lens Materials

The choice of the material has consequences on a variety of properties, such as the appearance, quality of vision, comfort (weight), transmission, safety, UV-absorption, and many more.

4.2.1 Refractive Index

In Sect. 2.2.1 we have already established that the refractive index is defined by the ratio of the velocity of light of a given frequency in vacuum c to the velocity of the same frequency in the refracting medium v.

Table 4.1 Refractive indices

Material	n_d	n_e
1.5	1.523	1.525
1.6	1.600	1.604
1.7	1.700	1.705
1.8	1.802	1.807
1.9	1.885	1.892

$$n = \frac{c}{v} \tag{4.1}$$

A lens with a higher refractive index material requires flatter curves (higher radii) to produce the required refractive power when compared to a lower refractive index material.

The refractive index n of an optical material is also dependent on the wavelength λ of light.

$$n = \frac{\lambda_c}{\lambda_v} \tag{4.2}$$

λ_c: Wavelength in vacuum

λ_v: Wavelength in medium

The Helium d-line ($\lambda = 587.56\,nm$) is used in the UK and the USA, whereas the Mercury e-line ($\lambda = 546.07\,nm$) is used in continental Europe. For instance, for Crown glass, the d-line produces a refractive index of $n_d = 1.523$, and the e-line gives a refractive index of $n_e = 1.525$; however, both materials are identical. Table 4.1 shows a few examples of refractive indices calculated for white light (d-line and e-line).

In Sect. 2.2.6.2 we have seen that the refractive power F of a curved optical surface is dependent on the refractive index n and the radius r of the surface.

$$F = \frac{n' - n}{r} \tag{4.3}$$

Hence, the refractive index n affects the thickness of a lens.

Remember

- The higher the refractive index n, the thinner the lens.

The relative curvature RC is used to indicate the degree of flattening achieved by the use of a higher refractive index material. The relative curvature RC predicts the reduction in edge thickness obtained and is used to predict the appearance of an ophthalmic lens. It can be used to determine the refractive index of an unknown lens. The relative curvature RC of a material is usually compared to Crown glass with a refractive index of $n = 1.523$.

$$RC = \frac{1.523 - 1}{n - 1} \tag{4.4}$$

Table 4.2 shows the thickness reduction (in %) for various refractive indices and relative curvatures RC.

Table 4.2 Refractive index, relative curvature & thickness reduction

Refractive index	Relative curvature (RC)	Thickness reduction (%)
1.6	0.87	13
1.7	0.75	25
1.8	0.65	35
1.9	0.58	42

4.2.2 Density and Weight

The density ρ is the ratio of mass m and volume V of a material $[kg/m^3]$.

$$\rho = \frac{m}{V} \tag{4.5}$$

Tables 4.3 and 4.4 show examples for the density ρ and refractive index n for various glass and plastic materials.

Remember
- The density of a material increases with increasing refractive index.

Table 4.3 Refractive index & density–glass

Material	n	ρ
1.5	1.523	2.54
1.6	1.600	2.63
1.7	1.701	3.21
1.8	1.802	3.65
1.9	1.885	3.99

Table 4.4 Refractive index & density–plastic

Material	n	ρ
CR39	1.49	1.30
Trivex	1.53	1.11
Tribid	1.60	1.23
Polycarbonate	1.59	1.20
1.6	1.60	1.30
1.67	1.67	1.36
1.74	1.74	1.46

4.2.3 Abbe Number

The term dispersion describes the dependence of the phase velocity v_P and its frequency λ. The phase velocity v_P is defined as the ratio of frequency f and time period T.

$$v_P = \frac{f}{T} \tag{4.6}$$

The Abbe number[1] or V-value V_d is a metric for the dispersion of a material and ultimately associated with the optical quality of a lens material. The Abbe number is defined as follows:

$$V_d = \frac{n_D - 1}{n_F - n_C} \tag{4.7}$$

where n_C, n_D and n_F denote the refractive indices of the material at the wavelengths of the Fraunhofer's C, D, and F spectral lines at $656.3nm$, $587.56nm$, and $486.1nm$, respectively. Table 4.5 shows the wavelengths and corresponding refractive indices that define the Abbe number.

Table 4.5 Fraunhofer spectral lines, refractive indices & wavelengths

Fraunhofer line	Wavelength [nm]	Refractive index n
Blue (Hydrogen)	$\lambda_F = 486.1$	$n_F = 1.505$
Yellow/orange (Sodium)	$\lambda_D = 587.56$	$n_D = 1.500$
Red (Hydrogen)	$\lambda_C = 656.3$	$n_C = 1.496$

[1]The Abbe number is named after the physicist Ernst Karl Abbe (1840–1905).

Remember

- Materials with a higher refractive index are often used to reduce lens volume.
- Materials with a higher refractive index are often associated with lower Abbe numbers.
- Materials with lower Abbe numbers can produce a reduction in visual quality.

- Low dispersion $V_d = 45$ and above
- Medium dispersion $V_d > 39 < 45$
- High dispersion $V_d < 39$

Tables 4.6 and 4.7 show various refractive indices and the corresponding Abbe numbers.

Table 4.6 Refractive index & Abbe number–glass

Medium	Refractive index	Abbe number
1.5	1.523	59
1.6	1.600	42
1.7	1.701	39
1.8	1.802	35
1.9	1.885	31

Table 4.7 Refractive index & Abbe number–plastic

Medium	Refractive index	Abbe number
CR39	1.50	59
Trivex	1.53	42
Eyas	1.60	39
Eynoa	1.67	35
Eyvia	1.74	31

4.2.4 Optical Aberrations

The principles of physical optics introduced in Chaps. 2 and 3 are based on the assumption that rays of light travel near the optic (principal) axis. For non-paraxial conditions, we have to consider optical aberrations. Optical aberration is a collective term for a variety of phenomena that have in common that light is spread out instead of being focused in a single point. There are many different optical aberrations. Here I will focus on chromatic, spherical and comatic aberrations (coma). Note that the astigmatism covered in Sects. 3.7 and 4.3 is a form of aberration, too.

4.2.4.1 Chromatic Aberration

In Sect. 4.2.1, we have established that the refractive index n of a material is dependent on the wavelength λ. Red light, for instance, has a lower wavelength than blue light (see Sect. 2.1). Given that the refractive power F of a lens is dependent on the refractive index (Eq. 2.16), it follows that blue light has a shorter focal length f' than red light. The aberrations related to colors are collectively referred to as chromatic aberrations, which can be divided into longitudinal (LCA) and transverse chromatic aberration (TCA). Figures 4.2 and 4.3 show illustrations of these chromatic aberrations.

$$LCA = \frac{F}{V_d} \tag{4.8}$$

LCA: Longitudinal chromatic aberration

F: Refractive power of lens

V_d: Abbe number

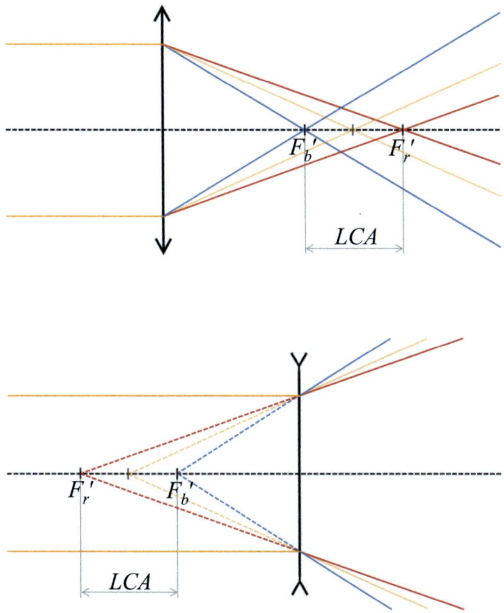

Fig. 4.2 The figure shows an illustration of longitudinal chromatic aberration (LCA) for a converging lens (top) and a diverging lens (bottom). F_b' denotes the second principal focus for blue, and F_r' for red light

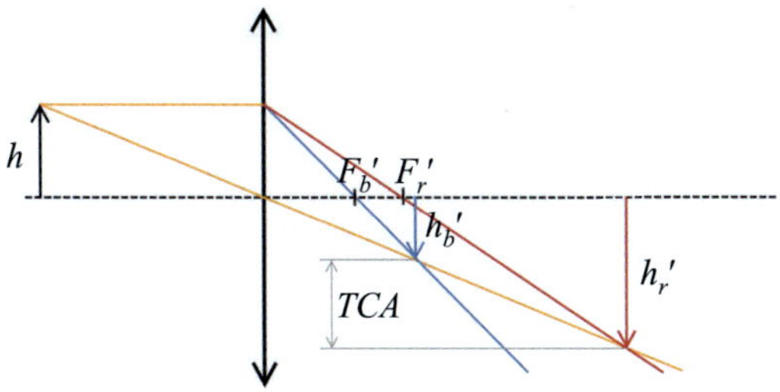

Fig. 4.3 The figure shows an illustration of transverse chromatic aberration (TCA). F_b' denotes the second principal focus for blue, and F_r' for red light

$$TCA = \frac{c \cdot F}{V_d} \tag{4.9}$$

TCA: Transverse chromatic aberration [$^{\Delta}$]

c: Decentration [cm] (see Sect. 4.5.2)

F: Refractive power of lens

V_d: Abbe number

Chromatic aberrations can affect the optical quality of the ophthalmic lens or lens system. Fine detail requires high contrast to be detectable. TCA degrades the contrast of the retinal image more than any other aberration. It is often stated that the average threshold value for TCA is 0.1^{Δ}. A TCA value $< 0.1^{\Delta}$ is unlikely to cause problems. However, TCA values $> 0.1^{\Delta}$ can significantly affect the visual acuity. Table 4.8 shows TCA values for various refractive powers and Abbe numbers.

Remember
Chromatic aberrations can be minimized by:

- Using high Abbe (V_d) number materials.
- The application of correct vertical centration and pantoscopic tilt.
- For low V_d materials, the optical centre of the lens should be placed on or close to the cente of the pupil.
- Sensible frame selection and small vertex distance.

Table 4.8 TCA value

F [D]	$V_D = 60$	$V_d = 40$	$V_d = 30$
–4.0	0.09^{Δ}	0.13^{Δ}	0.17^{Δ}
–6.0	0.13^{Δ}	0.19^{Δ}	0.26^{Δ}
–8.0	0.18^{Δ}	0.26^{Δ}	0.35^{Δ}
–10.00	0.22^{Δ}	0.33^{Δ}	0.44^{Δ}
–12.00	0.27^{Δ}	0.41^{Δ}	0.54^{Δ}

4.2.4.2 Spherical Aberration

The term spherical aberration describes the phenomenon that the refraction of paraxial rays is different from marginal rays. Similar to chromatic aberrations (Sect. 4.2.4.1), we can define longitudinal S_l and transverse spherical aberration S_t (Fig. 4.4).

$$S_l = k \cdot y^2 \tag{4.10}$$

$$S_t = \frac{k \cdot y^3}{f'_m} \tag{4.11}$$

S_l: longitudinal spherical aberration

S_t: transverse spherical aberration

y: Distance from optic axis

f'_m: Second focal length of marginal ray

k: constant

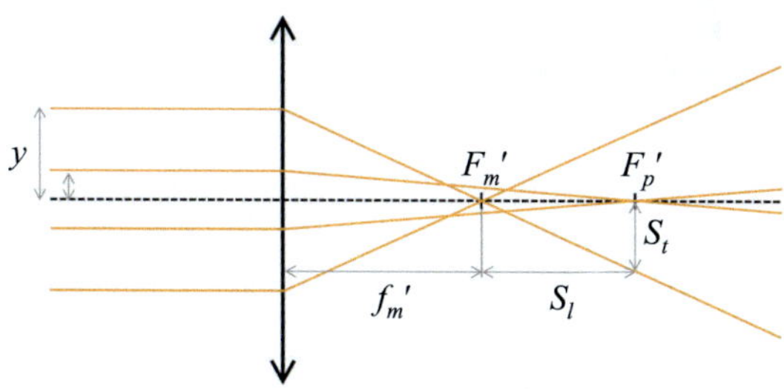

Fig. 4.4 The figure shows an illustration of longitudinal S_l and transverse spherical aberration S_t for a converging lens. F'_m denotes the second principal focus for marginal and F'_p for paraxial rays. f'_m is the second focal length of marginal rays

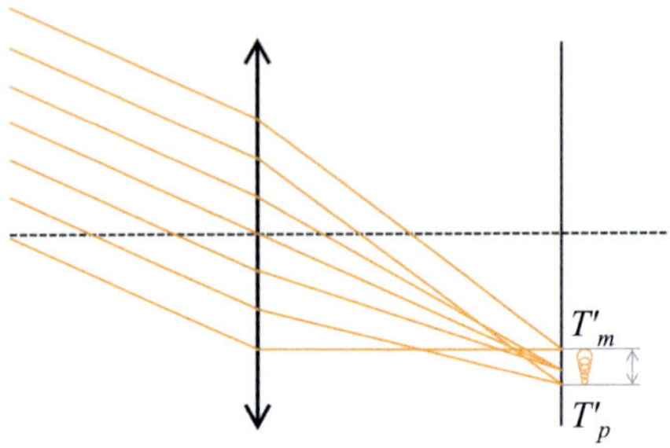

Fig. 4.5 The figure shows an illustration of the coma or comatic aberration, named after the comet-like distorsion instead of a point-like image

4.2.4.3 Coma

Coma or comatic aberration is a distortion of an image caused by specific optical designs or imperfections in the lens, which results in distorted off-axis point sources. They appear stretched or deformed, giving them a tail-like appearance similar to that of a comet. This is illustrated in Fig. 4.5.

4.2.5 Surface Reflectance

Surface reflectance and chromatic aberrations reduce the image contrast (for contrast see Sect. 7.2). An anti-reflection coating can be used to minimize surface reflections. However, an anti-reflection coating will not reduce LCA and TCA. The reflectivity R is a measure of the amount of surface reflection that occurs and is calculated according to:

$$R = \left(\frac{n' - n}{n' + n} \right)^2 \tag{4.12}$$

4.2.6 Summary

Remember

- Refractive index: The higher the refractive index, the thinner the lens.
- Relative curvature: The higher the refractive index, the lower the relative curvature. The lower the relative curvature, the thinner the lens.
- Density: The lower the density, the lighter the lens.
- Abbe number: The higher the Abbe number, the smaller is the chromatic aberration.
- UV cut-off: The higher the UV radiation cut-off, the safer to the eye.

4.3 Cylindrical Lenses

An astigmatic eye (Sect. 3.7) can be corrected with cylindrical lenses. A cylinder has two principal meridians, a flat

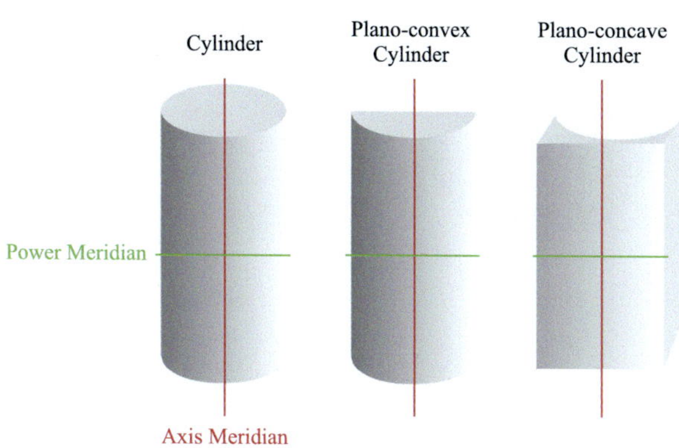

Fig. 4.6 The figure shows examples of cylinder lenses and the corresponding axis and power meridians

meridian referred to as the axis meridian and a steep meridian, referred to as the power meridian (Fig. 4.6).

In a plano-convex or plano-concave cylinder the axis meridian has a radius *r* of zero. Hence, according to Eq. 2.16, its refractive power is also zero; it's afocal.

4.3.1 Sphero-Cylindrical Lenses

A sphero-cylindrical lens is a combination of a spherical and a cylindrical lens. This combination is illustrated in Fig. 4.7.

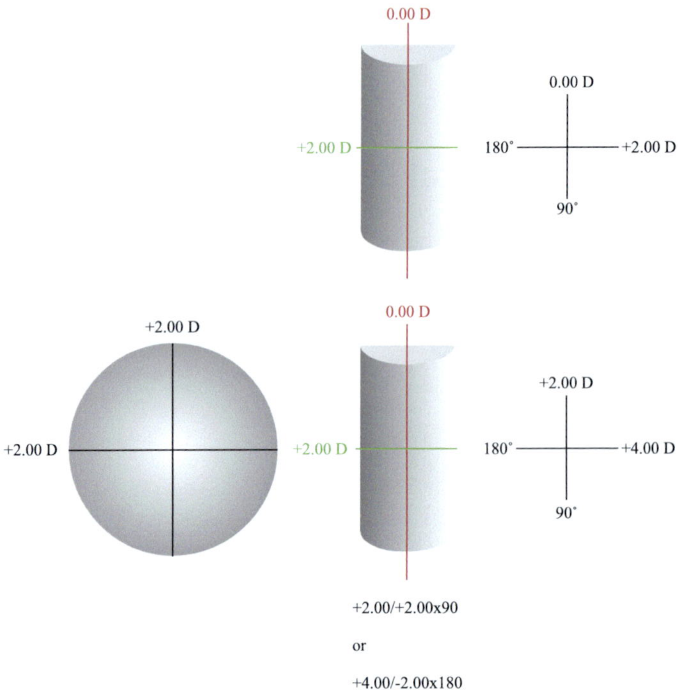

Fig. 4.7 The figure shows combinations of spherical and cylindrical lenses and the resulting power crosses and sphero-cylindrical combination

The standard notation for specifying a lens prescription is the sphere-cylinder prescription, which can be either positive or negative.

Remember
To transpose between a positive and negative sphere-cylinder form you follow the following rules.

1. $Sph + Cyl$
2. $Cyl \cdot (-1)$
3. $Axis + 90°$ (see example in Fig. 4.7)

4.4 Combination of Cylindrical Lenses

The power of two cylinders with the same axes is simply the sum of both (see Fig. 4.8).

A combination of cylinders where the axes are not 90° apart from each other is termed obliquely crossed cylinders. This scenario is depicted in Fig. 4.9.

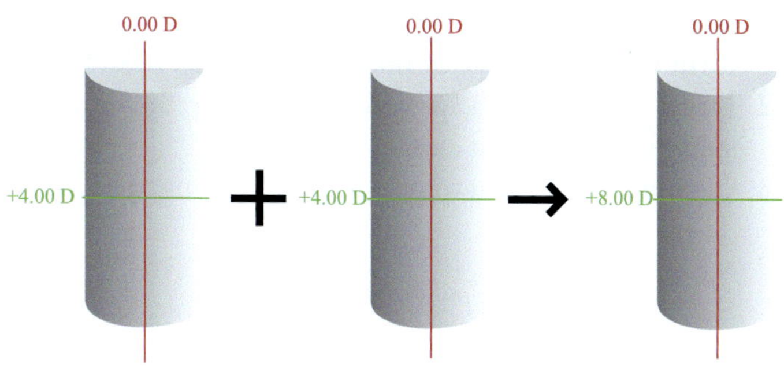

Fig. 4.8 Combination of cylinder lenses with the same axis

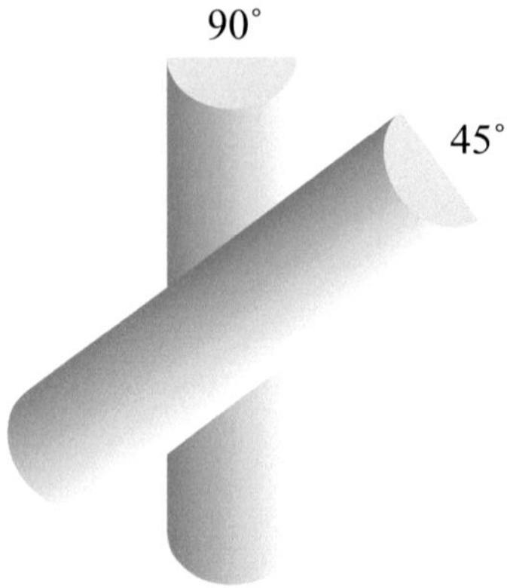

Fig. 4.9 Oblique crossed cylinders

There are various methods to determine the resulting power of obliquely crossed cylinders.

1. Graphical method
2. Astigmatic decomposition
3. Method by calculation

4.4.1 Graphical Solution

1. Convert the prescriptions into the same sph-cylinder form (either negative or positive); see Sect. 4.3.1).
2. Draw a table to help with calculating the resultant sphere, cylinder and axis.
3. Compute equivalent spheres E_{sph} according to Eq. 4.13.

$$E_{sph} = Sph + \frac{Cyl}{2} \tag{4.13}$$

4. Create a vector diagram to determine the resultant power.

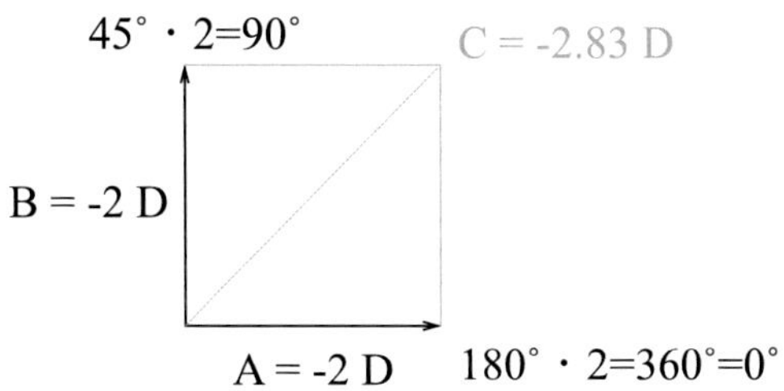

Fig. 4.10 Graphical method

a. Double the cylinder axis, but leave the cylinder power the same.
b. Draw the cylinder power to scale and the axis according to the doubled cylinder axis.
c. Draw the resultant vector.
d. Measure the length of the vector, which represents the power.
e. Measure the axis of the vector (Remember: This is twice the cylinder axis.).

5. Enter the new cylinder power and axis into the table.
6. Calculate the spherical equivalent of the resultant cylinder power and subtract this from the equivalent power calculated earlier. This is the new sphere power of the spherocylinder lens.

The example in Fig. 4.10 demonstrates the graphical method for the combination the following lenses:
Lens A: pl/-2.00x180
Lens B: pl/-2.00x45.

4.4.2 Astigmatic Decomposition

Any cylinder can be replaced by a combination of two cylinders with axes in specified directions. *C* is the resultant of

Table 4.9 Astigmatic decomposition

	M	C_0	C_{45}
Lens 1	M_1	C_0	C_{45}
Lens 2	M_2	C_0	C_{45}
$\sum$	$\sum M$	$\sum C_0$	$\sum C_{45}$

two components, C_0 along 0° (180°) and C_{45} along 45°. The spherical element is the mean sphere M (Table 4.9).

Lens 1

$$C_0 = C_1 \cdot cos(2 \cdot cyl_1) \tag{4.14}$$

$$C_{45} = C_1 \cdot sin(2 \cdot cyl_1) \tag{4.15}$$

$$M_1 = S_1 + \frac{C_1}{2} \tag{4.16}$$

Lens B

$$C_0 = C_2 \cdot cos(2 \cdot cyl_2) \tag{4.17}$$

$$C_{45} = C_2 \cdot sin(2 \cdot cyl_2) \tag{4.18}$$

$$M_2 = S_2 + \frac{C_2}{2} \tag{4.19}$$

$$C_R = \pm\sqrt{\sum C_0^2 + \sum C_{45}^2} \tag{4.20}$$

$$S_{total} = \sum M - (\frac{C_R}{2}) \tag{4.21}$$

$$\theta = arctan\left(\frac{C_R - \sum C_0}{\sum C_{45}}\right) \tag{4.22}$$

4.4.3 Calculation Method

1. Convert the prescriptions into the same sph-cylinder form (either negative or positive); see Sect. 4.3.1).
2. Find the difference between the two axes. **Assumption:** $\theta_{cyl_1} < \theta_{cyl_2}$
3. Calculate the axis of the new cylinder.
4. Calculate the new cylinder axis and add γ to the first cylinder axis.
5. Find the sphere power S caused by the obliquely crossed cylinder.
6. Find the new cylindrical power C.
7. Find the total sphere power S_{total} by adding the sphere powers from the original lenses to the sphere power resulting from the cross cylinder.

$$\alpha = \theta_{cyl_2} - \theta_{cyl_1} \tag{4.23}$$

$$\gamma = \frac{atan\left(\frac{|C_2|sin2\alpha}{|C_1|+|C_2|cos2\alpha}\right)}{2} \tag{4.24}$$

$$\theta_{cyl} = \gamma + \theta_{cyl_1} \tag{4.25}$$

$$S = C_1 \cdot sin(\gamma)^2 + C_2 \cdot sin(\alpha - \gamma)^2 \tag{4.26}$$

$$C_R = C_1 + C_2 - 2S \tag{4.27}$$

$$S_{total} = S + S_1 + S_2 \tag{4.28}$$

C_1: Power of cylinder of lens 1

C_2: Power of cylinder of lens 2

C_R: Resulting cylinder

γ: Difference to δ_{cyl_1}

θ_{cyl_1}: Cylinder axis of lens 1

θ_{cyl_2}: Cylinder axis of lens 2

S: Sphere power caused by the obliquely crossed cylinder

α: Difference between the two cylinder axes

θ_{cyl}: Resulting cylinder axis

S_{total}: Total sphere power

4.5 Prisms as Ophthalmic Lenses

We have already established the optical properties of prisms in Sect. 2.2.5. Ophthalmic prisms tend to have an apical angle $\alpha < 10°$ (see Fig. 2.4). Prisms in optometric practice are used to correct heterophorias (muscle imbalances), strabismus (squint), and to improve the appearance of progressive power lenses (prism thinning). Figure 4.11 shows an illustration of the prismatic deviation caused by a prism with a particular base direction.

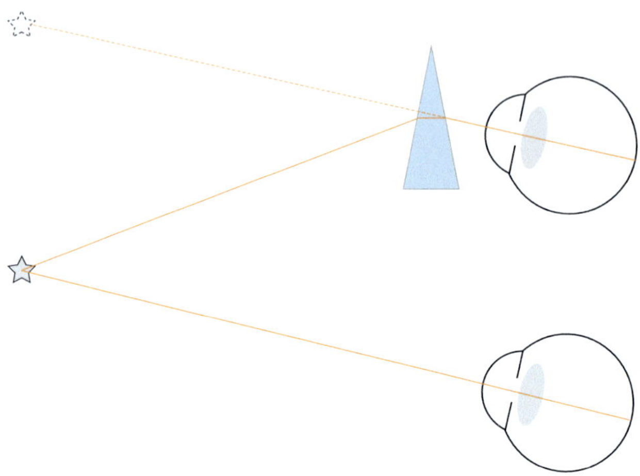

Fig. 4.11 Prismatic effect

4.5.1 Prism Diopter

For a prism with an apical angle α, the angle of deviation δ can be calculated according to:

$$\delta = (n - 1) \cdot \alpha \tag{4.29}$$

The prism diopters P [$^{cm}/_{m}$ or ($^{\Delta}$)] is defined as the number of centimeters an image is displaced at a distance of one meter (x). This is shown in Fig. 4.12.

$$P = \frac{D}{x} \quad [^{\Delta}] \tag{4.30}$$

δ: Angle of deviation

n: Refractive index of prism

α: Apical angle of prism

Remember

- The prismatic effect is measured in prism diopters.
- The prism diopter is the amout of prism deviation in centimetres at a distance of $1m$.
- The unit of the prism diopter is $^{cm}/_{m}$; often symbolized as $^{\Delta}$.

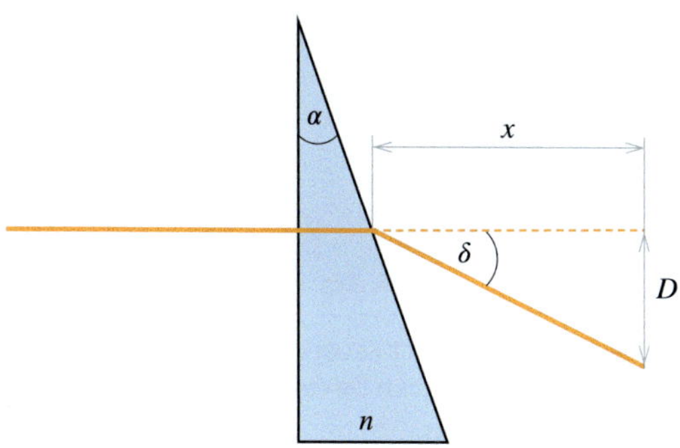

Fig. 4.12 Prism deviation

4.5.2 Prentice's Rule

The prismatic effect P of a lens at any given point can be calculated by the following equation:

$$P = c \cdot F \tag{4.31}$$

P: Prism power [$^{\Delta}$]

c: Decentration (distance of optical center [cm])

F: Lens power [D])

This is referred to as Prentice's rule, named after Charles F. Prentice (Fig. 4.13).

4.5.3 Prism Notation

The direction of a prism is described by the direction of the base in relation to the eye. Figure 4.14 shows the corresponding terminology. The prismatic power of a lens can be

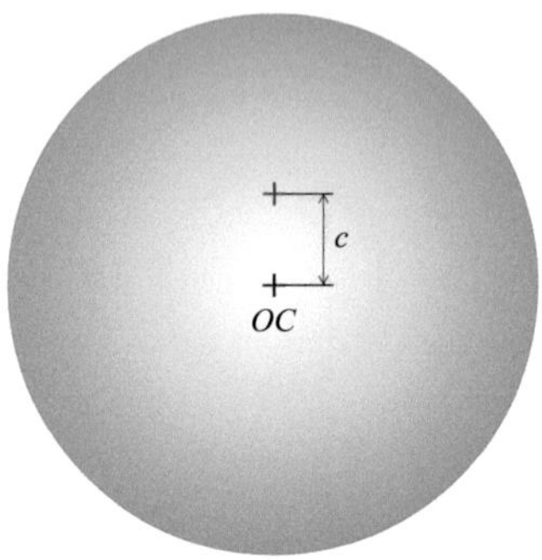

Fig. 4.13 The prismatic effect caused by a decentration c [cm] from the optical center point OC can be calculated according to the Prentice rule (Eq. 4.5.2)

described by the horizontal and vertical prismatic power as separate components. This format is known as the resolving prism power (e.g. 5^{Δ} down $3^{\Delta} in$). Alternatively, one can express the prismatic power as a single power in a particular meridian. This format is known as the compounding prism power (e.g., 5.83^{Δ} down & in along 121°). We can resolve the vertical and horizontal prismatic power into a compounding prism power using the Pythagorean theorem and trigonometry to calculate the orientation of a prism (see Chap. 1).

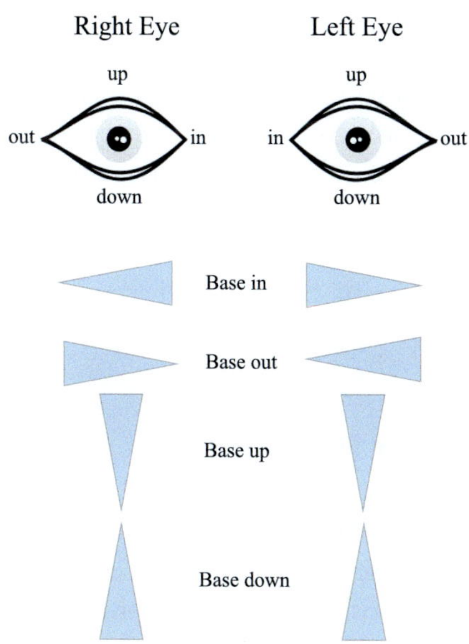

Fig. 4.14 Prism notation

Remember

- Base in + Base in ⟶ summative effect
- Base out + Base out ⟶ summative effect

- Base in + Base out ⟶ subtractive effect
- Base up + Base up ⟶ subtractive effect
- Base down + Base down ⟶ subtractive effect
- Base down + Base up ⟶ summative effect

4.6 Exercises

1. What is the sphero-cylindrical power for the following combination of obliquely crossed cylinders?
   Lens A: $-3.50/-4.00x45°$
   Lens B: $-2.50/-1.50x90°$
   Use the astigmatic decomposition method.
2. What is the sphero-cylindrical power for the following combination of obliquely crossed cylinders?
   Lens A: $-1.00/-2.00x20°$
   Lens B: $-2.50/-3.00x80°$
   Use the astigmatic calculation method.

4.7 Further Reading

- Bennett AG, Rabbetts RB. Bennett and Rabbetts' clinical visual optics. Elsevier Health Sciences; 1998.
- Brooks CW, Borish I. System for ophthalmic dispensing-e-book. Elsevier Health Sciences; 2006.
- Keating MP. Geometric, physical, and visual optics. Elsevier Health Sciences; 1988.
- Keirl A, Christie C, editors. Clinical optics and refraction: A guide for optometrists, contact lens opticians and

dispensing opticians. Butterworth Heinemann, Elsevier Health Sciences; 2007.

- Tunnacliffe AH. Introduction to visual optics. London: Association of british dispensing opticians; 1993.

5

Optical Instruments

The principles of geometric and physical optics covered in Chaps. 2 and 3 are at the heart of most optical instruments that are utilized for examinations and diagnostic purposes in optometric and ophthalmic practice. In the following chapter, I will summarize some of the most common optical instruments, their physical properties and utilization.

5.1 Basics

5.1.1 Depth of Focus

The depth of focus d_f of a lens or lens system is defined as the axial range over which the image plane can be moved without noticeable difference in the image definition. Note that the depth of focus is dependent on the aperture size as illustrated in Fig. 5.1.

G. Schmidtmann, *Clinical Vision Science*, https://doi.org/10.1007/978-3-031-83321-2_5

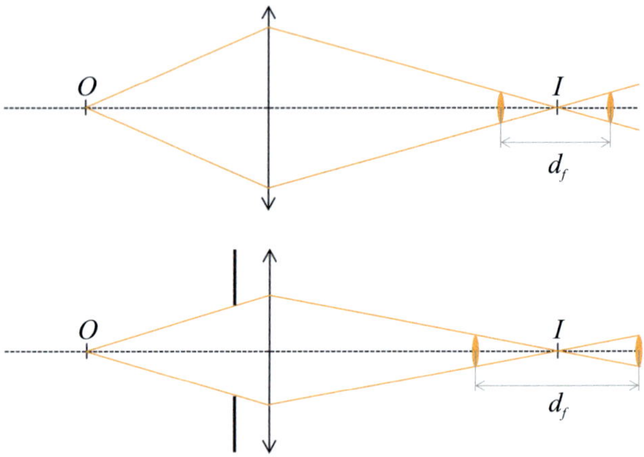

Fig. 5.1 The figure shows the depth of focus d_f for two different apertures. The maxiumum size of the undetectable blur circle is illustrated by the orange ellipses

5.1.2 Depth of Field

The depth of field d_{fd} of a lens or lens system is defined as the distance between the axial positions of an object which produces a blur disc of equal size without noticeable difference in the image definition (see Fig. 5.2). Note, that similar to the depth of focus, the depth of field is also dependent on the aperture size.

Remember
- The depth of focus and depth of field are inversely proportional to the size of the aperture.
- In other words, the depth of focus and depth of field increase with decreasing aperture size and vice versa.

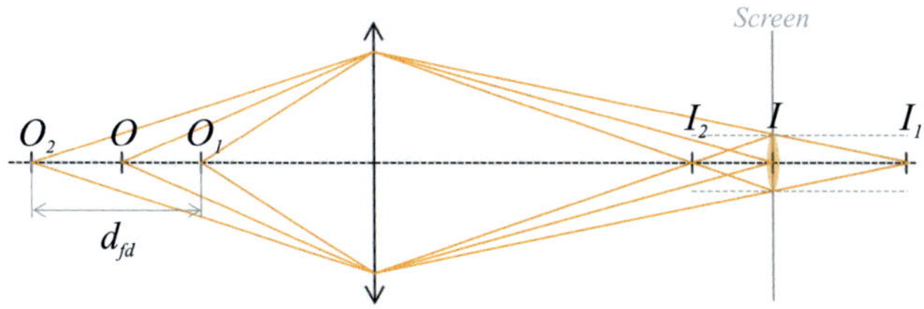

Fig. 5.2 The figure shows the depth of field d_{fd}. Note that the object at position 1 (O_1) and position 2 (O_2) produce a blur disc (orange ellipse) of the same size

5.2 Magnification

The term magnification refers to the process of increasing the apparent size (perceived, not physical) of an object. Many optical instruments utilize magnification (e.g., telescope, microscope, magnifying glass, etc.).

Remember

An image magnification can be achieved by (Fig. 5.3):

- Decreasing the viewing distance (Fig. 5.3B).
- Increasing the object size (Fig. 5.3C).
- Increasing the angular subtense of α' by a lens with a positive refractive power (Fig. 5.3D).

The magnification can be calculated according to:

$$M = \frac{h'}{h} = \frac{l'}{l} = \frac{L}{L'} \tag{5.1}$$

h: Object size

h': Image size

L: Vergence in (incident vergence) $[D]$

L': Vergence out (exit vergence) $[D]$

l: Distance to object $[m]$

l': Distance to image $[m]$

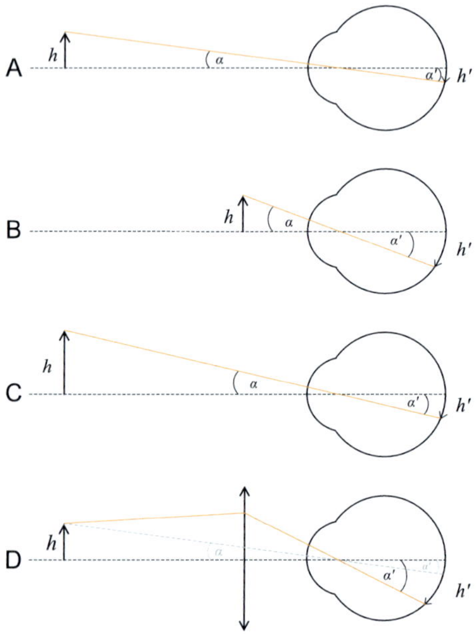

Fig. 5.3 Methods for image magnification

5.2.1 Angular Magnification

The angular magnification M_a relates the angle subtended by the unaided eye α with the angle subtended by the image produced by a lens or lens system β.

$$M_a = \frac{\beta}{\alpha} \tag{5.2}$$

M_a: Angular magnification

α: Angle subtended at unaided eye by object at least distance of distinct vision (Standard: $0.25m$)

β: Angle subtended at eye by image produced by lens

5.2.2 Spectacle Magnification

The term spectacle magnification (M_s) describes the ratio of corrected (h'_{cc}) and uncorrected (h'_{sc}) retinal image size.

$$M_s = \frac{h'_{cc}}{h'_{sc}} \tag{5.3}$$

For thin lenses, the spectacle magnification can be calculated according to the following equation.

$$M_s = \frac{1}{1 - (d \cdot F_{sp})} \tag{5.4}$$

M_s: Spectacle magnification

F_{sp}: Spectacle lens power $[D]$

d: Vertex distance $[m]$

5.3 Telescopes

Figure 5.4 shows ray diagrams for the two most common types of telescopes, the astronomical (top) and Galilean telescope (bottom). The astronomical telescope is also referred to Keplerian telescope.[1]

Remember

- The astronomical telescope (Keplerian telescope) consists of two converging (plus) lenses.
- The Galilean telescope consists of a positive objective and a negative eyepiece (ocular).

[1]The Keplerian telescope is named after the astronomer and mathematician Johannes Kepler (1571–1630). The Galilean telescope is named after Galileo Galilei (1564–1642).

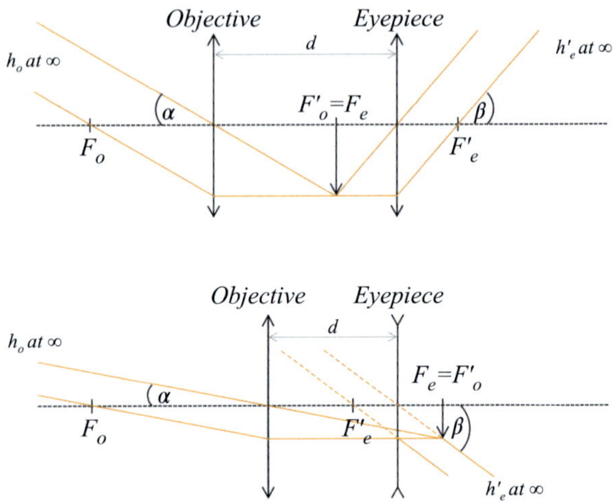

Fig. 5.4 The figure shows ray diagrams for an astronomical (also Keplerian, top) and a Galilean telescope (bottom)

The magnification M_t of telescopes can be calculated according to:

$$M_t = -\frac{F_e}{F_o} = -\frac{f_o}{f_e'} \tag{5.5}$$

F_e: Power of eyepiece

f_e: Focal length of eyepiece

F_o: Power of objective

f_o: Focal length of objective

5.4 Simple Magnifier (Loupe)

If the image is formed at infinity as shown in Fig. 5.5, the magnification is referred to as the nominal magnification

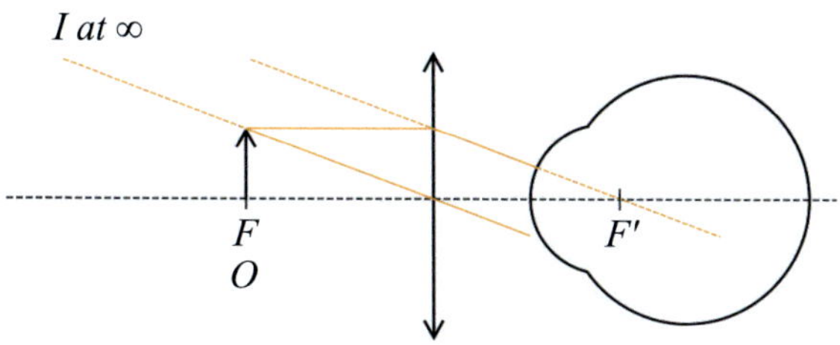

Fig. 5.5 The figure shows a simple magnifier where the object is located in the primary focal point. Hence, the image is formed at infinity

M_{nom}.

$$M_{nom} = \frac{F}{4} \tag{5.6}$$

The maximum magnification M_{max} of a simple magnifier is calculated as follows.

$$M_{max} = 1 + \frac{F}{4} \tag{5.7}$$

5.5 Microscope

Figure 5.6 shows the ray diagram for a microscope.

5.6 Focimeter

The focimeter is an instrument that can be used to measure the vertex power (back or front vertex power) of a lens. It can also be utilized to find the orientation of the cylinder axis, the location the optical center of a lens, and to determine the prismatic power at any point of a lens.

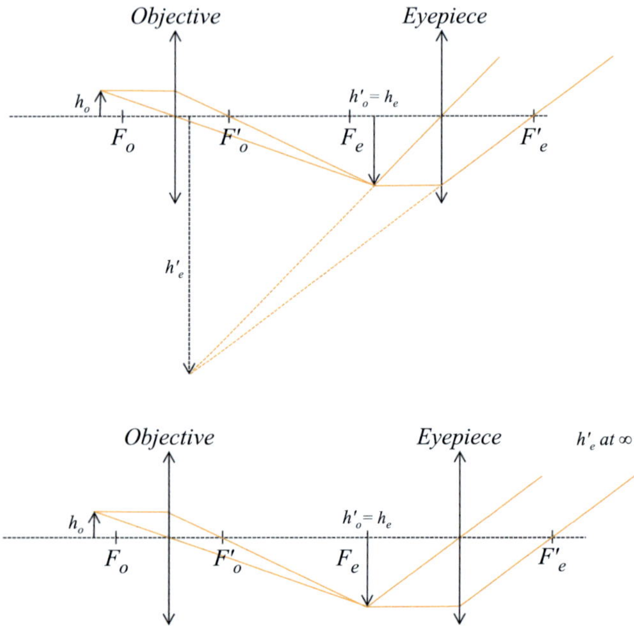

Fig. 5.6 The figure shows ray diagrams of a microscope for two different object locations

5.6.1 Optical Features of the Focimeter

The focimeter consists of the following parts.

- Collimator–Standard lens (F_O around $+25.00D$ achromatic doublet)
- Movable target to produce parallel light
- Lens rest at the second principal focus

- Telescope–designed to focus parallel light (eye-piece needs adjusting for the individual using the instrument). The image of the target (when focused) will be seen in the same plane as the graticule (see Sect. 5.3)

5.6.2 Optical Principles of the Focimeter

With no lens in position, the target reads zero when it is at the first principal focus of F_O. Since the emergent light from the collimator is parallel under these circumstances, the target image will be clear and in focus and in the same plane as the graticule. The lens under test, when placed on the lens rest, lies at the second principal focus of the standard lens (F_O'). The target is moved by using the focusing wheel until the target image is in focus. This will also place the image of the target at the test lens second principal focus. The amount of target movement is linearly proportional to the focal length (and hence the power) of the lens under test. The focusing wheel can therefore be calibrated in diopters (usually $0.12D$) (Fig. 5.7).

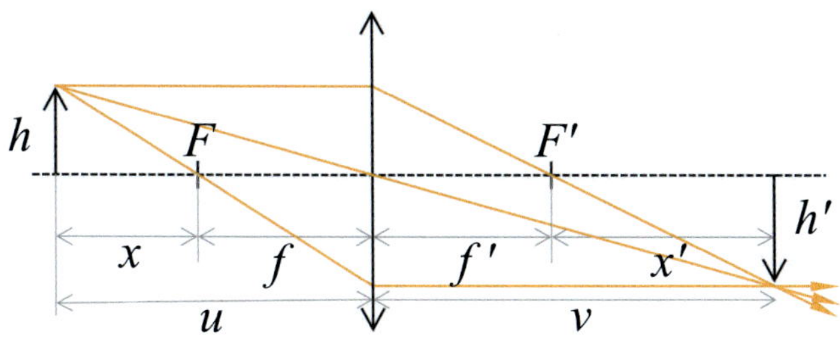

Fig. 5.7 Newton relation

f: First principal focal length
f': Second principal focal length
x: Extra-focal object distance
x': Extra-focal image distance

Newton's equation:

$$x \cdot x' = f \cdot f' \tag{5.8}$$

For a lens in air:

$$x \cdot x' = -f_2' \tag{5.9}$$

With a lens placed on the lens rest:

$$x \cdot f_v' = f_o'^2 \tag{5.10}$$

and

$$x \cdot F_v = F_o^2 \tag{5.11}$$

The movement of the target per diopter of the power of the lens under test is linear (Fig. 5.8). If the standard lens power was $+25.00D$ then the movement of the target would be $1.6mm$. In order to measure lens powers in the range

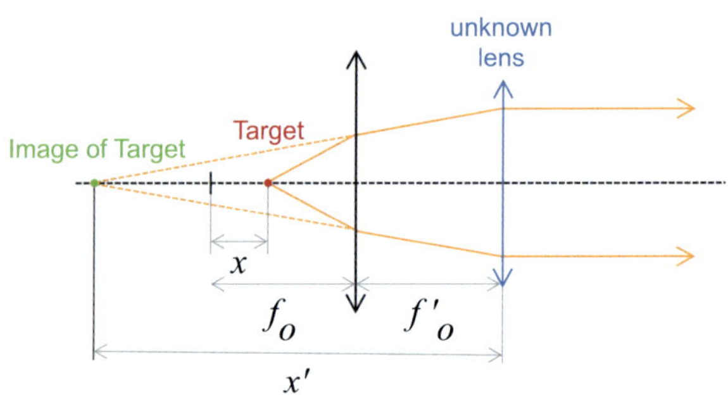

Fig. 5.8 Focimeter principle

$+20.00D$ to $-20.00D$ the total travel of the target needs to be $40 \cdot 1.6 = 64mm$.

5.6.3 Usage of Focimeter

The following section will provide a step-by-step guide of focimetry of spherical and sphero-cylindrical lenses. All figures below show illustrations of the European Dot Target Focimeter (left) and the US Line Target Focimeter (right). In order to measure the power of an ophthalmic lens, you have to place the back surface of the lens on the lens rest and hold it in place using the stage and spring-loaded holder. Make sure the dotting mechanism is in its resting position. The instrument will then be measuring the back vertex power of the lens. If you want to measure the front vertex power, you will have to place the front surface on the lens rest–this is sometimes required for determining the Addition in multifocal lenses.

5.6.4 Focimetry of Spherical Lenses–Procedure

For a spherical lens, there will be only one position of the focusing wheel where the image (target) is focused. Ideally, the lens should be adjusted so that the target is in the middle of the graticule.

1. Focus the graticule (i.e., protractor) by adjusting the eyepiece of the focimeter.
2. The dot target (green in figures below) should be centered and focused when the scale is at $0.00D$ (otherwise the focimeter has to be calibrated).

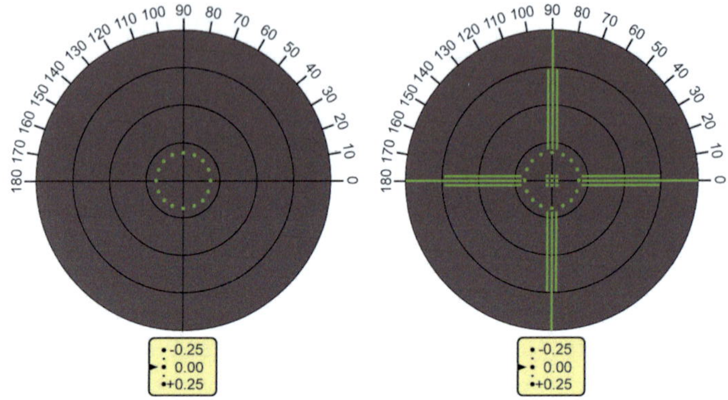

3. Place the back surface of the lens on the lens rest and fixate it with the spring-loaded holder.
4. Rotate the power focusing wheel to its maximum (either + or –).
5. The dot / line target will be blurry and occur at a random position on the graticule.

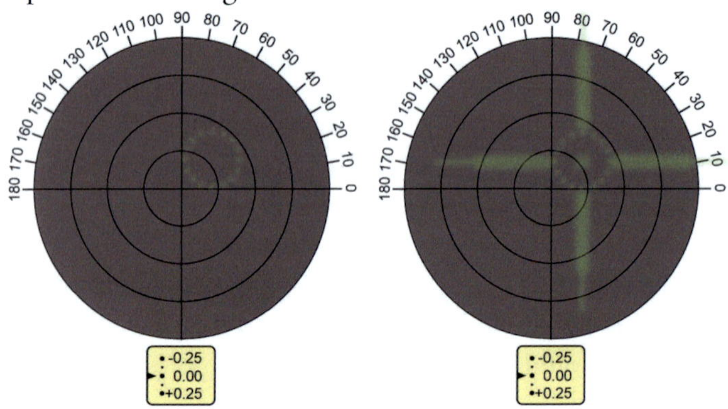

6. Try to move the target into approximately the center of the graticule.

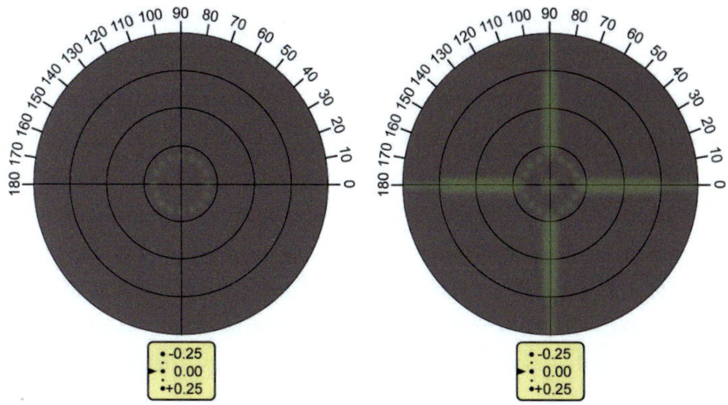

7. Turn the power wheel until the target appears focused.
8. Adjust the lens horizontally and vertically to position the target exactly in the middle of the graticule.

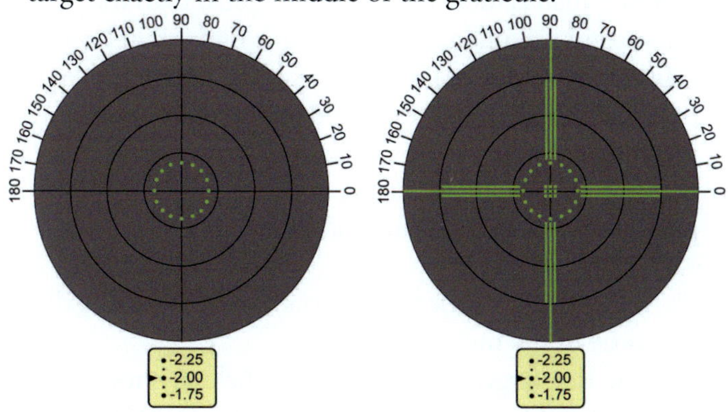

9. Read off the power from the scale ($-2.00D$ in the example).
10. Hence, the power of the lens is $-2.00DS$ (sphere only).
11. Having recorded the result, you can at this stage employ the dotting mechanism to place ink dots (usually three), where the central dot indicates the optical center of the test lens. The center of the graticule representes the point on the lens where there is no prismatic effect (optical center).

5.6.5 Focimetry of Sphero-Cylindrical Lenses–Procedure

A sphero-cylindrical lens has two principal meridians (i.e., powers), which are perpendicular (90°) to each other (see Sect. 4.301). Each meridian produces orthogonal line images (see Sect. 3.7). As a consequence, the individual dots of the target will appear as lines (target lines) with a particular axis. The axes of both meridians are perpendicular to each other. There is often confusion about what the cylinder of a sphero-cylindrical lens is and whether it is a plus or minus cylinder. The cylinder power is simply the difference between the power of the two meridians in D. Hence, if the power of the first meridian is more positive (more plus) than the power of the second meridian, the resulting cylinder will be a minus cylinder. Conversely, if the power of the first meridian is less positive (more minus) compared to the second meridian, the resulting cylinder is a plus cylinder. You can choose each of these meridians as the sphere and express your results in a plus–or minus cylinder notation.

1. Focus the graticule (i.e., protractor) by adjusting the eyepiece of the focimeter.
2. The dot target (green in figures below) should be centered and focused when the scale is at $0.00D$ (otherwise the focimeter has to be calibrated).

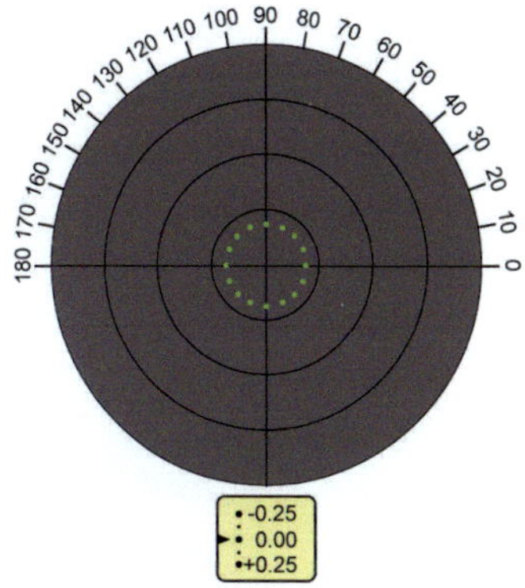

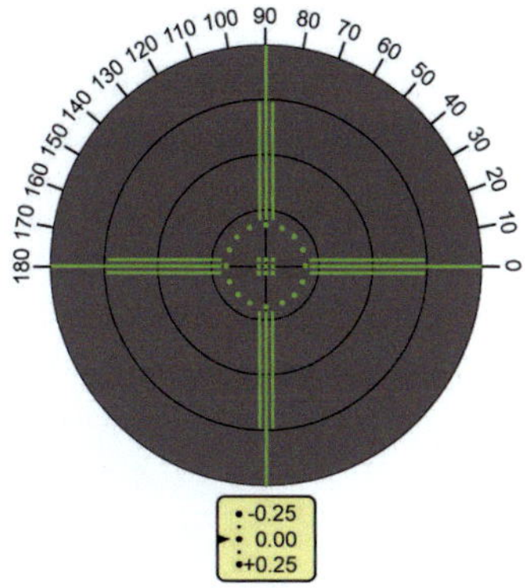

3. Place the back surface of the lens on the lens rest and fixate it with the spring-loaded holder.
4. The target will be blurry and occur at a random position on the graticule.

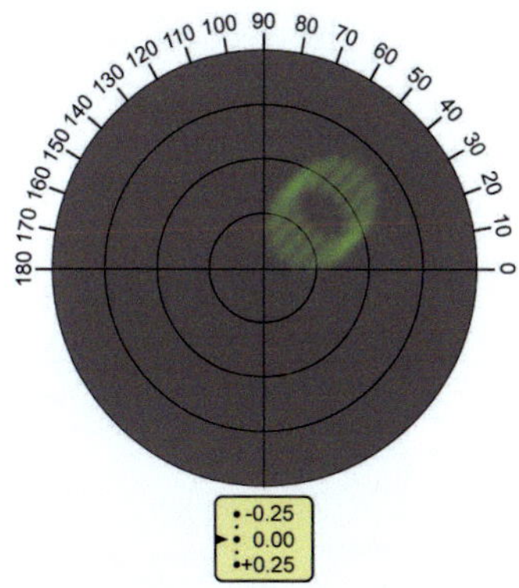

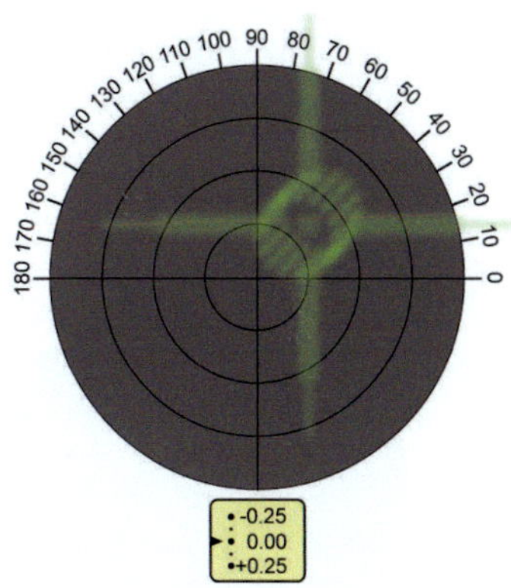

5. Try to move the target into approximately the center of the graticule.
6. For the US Line Target Focimeter, turn the axis wheel so that the longer lines are parallel to the shorter target lines (this is indicated by the arrow in the illustration below).

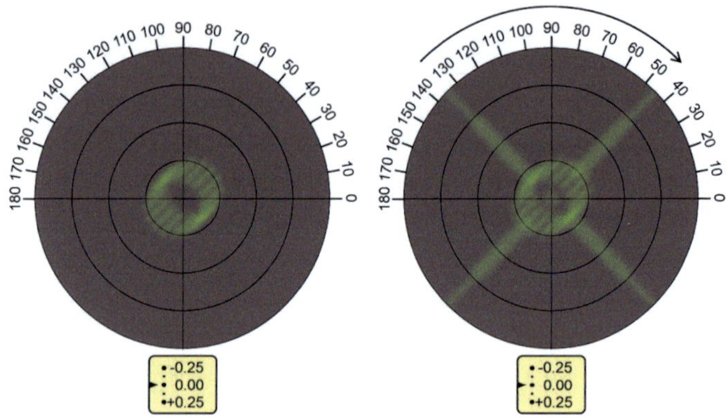

7. Turn the power wheel until the target appears focused (Meridian I).
8. Adjust the lens horizontally and vertically to position the target exactly in the middle of the graticule.
9. Turn the power wheel to focus the second meridian (Meridian II).
10. Switch back and forth between both meridians in order to center the target on the graticule.

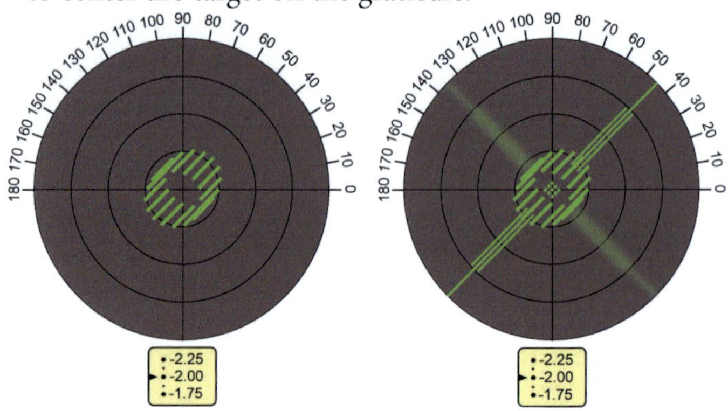

11. Choose one of the two meridians as your sphere.
12. Read off the power from the scale (Power Meridian I = $-2.00D$ in the example above).

13. Read off the axis of this meridian by using the protractor (Axis of Meridian I = 45° in exampe above).

Meridian	Power	Axis
I	$-2.00D$	45°
II		

14. Turn the power wheel to the second meridian (Meridian II).
15. Read off the power from the scale (Power Meridian II = $-4.00D$ in the example above).
16. Read off the axis of this meridian by using the protractor (Axis of Meridian II = 135° in exampe above).

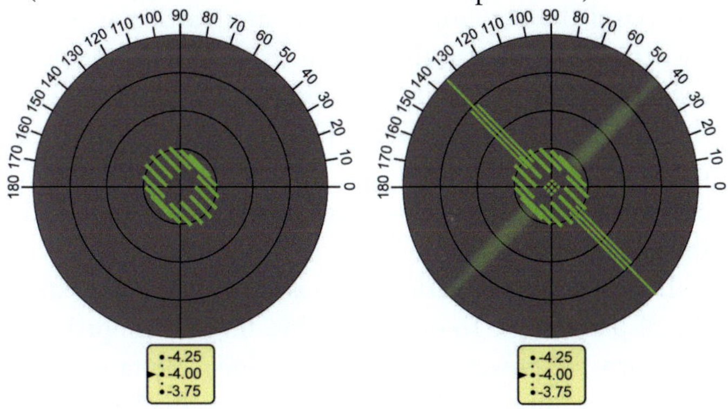

Meridian	Power	Axis
I	$-2.00D$	45°
II	$-4.00D$	135°

17. Meridian I is the Sphere.
18. The difference between Meridian I and Meridian II is the cylinder.
19. The Axis of Meridian II is the axis of the cylinder.
    $-2.00DS$ / $-2.00DC$ x 135°

Alternatively,

20. Meridian II is the Sphere.
21. The difference between Meridian II and Meridian I is the cylinder.
22. The Axis of Meridian I is the axis of the cylinder.
$-4.00DS$ / $+2.00DC$ x 45°

5.6.5.1 Focimetry of Prisms

To record the amount of prism at any particular point on the lens (other than at the optical center), the graticule consists of a tangent scale in 1^{Δ} divisions. The displacement of the target can be estimated either in vertical or horizontal components, or as a resultant. In order to specify base in or out, we need to know whether the test lens is intended for the left or right eye.

If the lens is astigmatic, then it is more difficult to estimate the displacement. To overcome this, find the dioptric mean and turn the power wheel to this value. The target will be blurry, but importantly, this blur will be circular (since this will be the circle of least confusion of the astigmatic pencil). It is then much easier to estimate the center of this blur circle and its displacement on the tangent scale.

5.6.6 Prism Base Direction

Figure 5.9 illustrates the prism base positions in the focimeter.

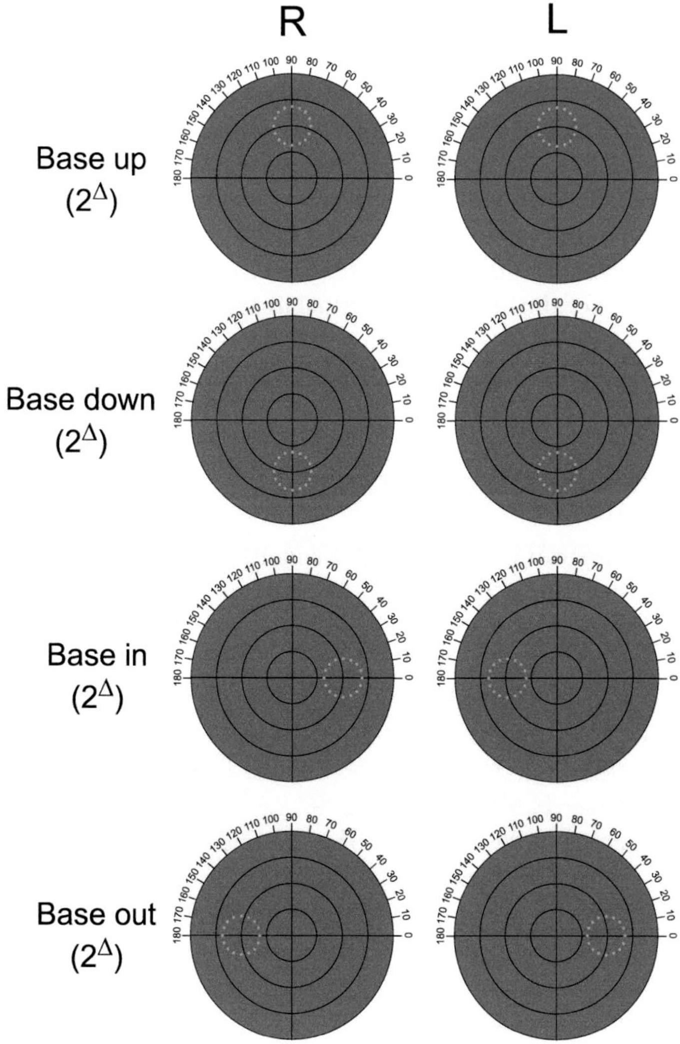

Fig. 5.9 Prism base positions

5.7 Exercises

1. Calculate the size of the retinal image of an object with a height of 30cm located at a distance of 1 m away from a schematic reduced eye with an axial length of 22mm.
2. Calculate the size of the retinal image in an eye which has been corrected with a $-12.00D$ spectacle lens positioned at a distance of 10mm in front of the eye, if the size of the uncorrected retinal image is 0.5mm? Assume a thin lens.

5.8 Further Reading

- Bennett AG, Rabbetts RB. Bennett and Rabbetts' clinical visual optics. Elsevier Health Sciences; 1998.
- Brooks CW, Borish I. System for ophthalmic dispensing-e-book. Elsevier Health Sciences; 2006.
- Freeman MH, Hull CC. Optics. 11th Edition. Butterworth Heinemann. 2003.
- Jackson AJ, Wolffsohn JS, editors. Low vision manual. Elsevier Health Sciences; 2007.
- Keating MP. Geometric, physical, and visual optics. Elsevier Health Sciences; 1988.
- Keirl A, Christie C, editors. Clinical optics and refraction: A guide for optometrists, contact lens opticians and dispensing opticians. Butterworth Heinemann, Elsevier Health Sciences; 2007.
- Lahiri, A. Basic Optics: Principles and Concepts., Elsevier Science. 2016.
- Tunnacliffe AH. Introduction to visual optics. London: Association of british dispensing opticians; 1993.

6

Photometry

The study of the measurement of light in terms of the visual response (either the eye or optical instruments, e.g., light meter) is referred to as photometry. This chapter seeks to highlight the most important units, measurements and numbers in photometry. The content of this chapter is not necessarily the subject of clinical optometry or ophthalmology; however, you might encounter some of the units and measurements in the user manuals of common clinical tests, e.g., color vision tests, or visual acuity charts.

6.1 Angular Measures

6.1.1 Flat Angles

The radian is the angle subtended at the centre of a circle by an arc equal to its radius (Fig. 6.1). A complete angle (360°) in radians, surrounding a point would be given by 2π (see Fig. 1.1).

G. Schmidtmann, *Clinical Vision Science*,
https://doi.org/10.1007/978-3-031-83321-2_6

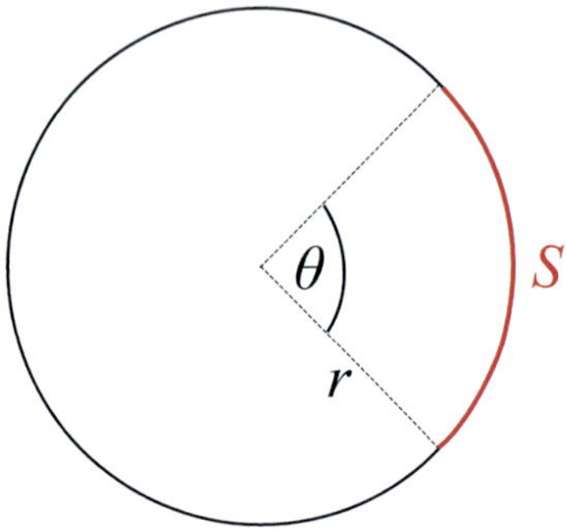

Fig. 6.1 Definition radian

$$\theta = \frac{S}{r} \tag{6.1}$$

S: Arc length

r: Radius

6.1.2 Solid Angle

A light source usually emits light in all directions. It is therefore important to consider the entire space around the light source. The space around a light source can be divided into solid angles, which are measured in steradians. This is illustrated in Fig. 6.2.

The solid anlge (steradian) ω is given by:

$$\omega = \frac{A}{r^2} \tag{6.2}$$

ω: Solid angle [steradian]

A: Spherical surface area

r: Radius of the sphere

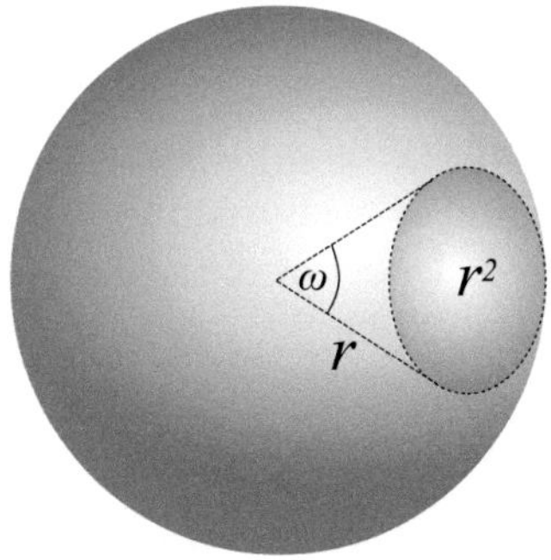

Fig. 6.2 Definition steradian

A complete solid angle in steradian, surrounding a point is 4π.

6.2 Light Intensity

In general terms, any lighting system and the illuminated environment can be characterized by four defined terms:

1. The intensity of the source.
2. The rate at which light energy radiates from the light source in a specified direction.
3. The amount of light falling on a unit surface area.
4. The amount of light reflected from or emitted by a unit area of surface in a given direction.

6.2.1 Luminous Intensity

The luminous intensity I_v is the strength of the source in a given direction and is measured in candela. One candela cd is $1/60$ of I_v from 1 cm^2 of the surface of platinum at its freezing point (ca. $1,773°C$).

$$I_v = \frac{\Phi}{\omega} \tag{6.3}$$

I_v: luminous intensity

Φ: luminous flux

ω: Solid angle [Steradian]

6.2.2 Luminous Flux

The luminous flux Φ is the rate of the flow of light energy from a point source.

$$\Phi = \omega \cdot I_v \tag{6.4}$$

where ω is the solid angle into which the light flows from the point source of intensity I_v. The unit of flux is Lumen. Table 6.1 shows luminous intensities for some common light sources.

Table 6.1 Luminous intensity of some common sources

Source	Luminous intensity [cd]
Candle	~ 1
100 Watt lamp	~ 120
Sun	$\sim 10^{27}$

Table 6.2 Illuminance [lux][1]

Source	Illuminance [lux]
Direct bright sunlight	10^5
Clear daylight	10^4
Full moon	10^{-1}
Clear night without moon	10^{-3}

6.2.3 Illuminance

The illuminance E_v is the measure of the luminous flux density at a point on an illuminated surface and is measured in lux.

$$E_v = \frac{\Phi}{A} \tag{6.5}$$

$$\left[\frac{Lumen}{m^2} = lux\right] \tag{6.6}$$

Typical (recommended) levels of illuminance are summarized in Table 6.2.

6.2.4 Luminance

The luminance L_v is the amount of light per unit area emitted or reflected in a given direction by a surface $[cd/m^2]$. The luminance of some objects is summarized in Table 6.3.

Table 6.3 Luminance $[cd/m^2]$ [1]

Source	Luminance $[cd/m^2]$
Surface of the sun	$1.6 \cdot 10^9$
Arc lamp	$3.0 \cdot 10^8$
Candle	$2.0 \cdot 10^6$
Clear blue sky	$1.0 \cdot 10^4$
Moon	$2.6 \cdot 10^3$
Moonless clear night	$1.0 \cdot 10^{-3}$

6.3 Light Intensity Laws

6.3.1 Inverse Square Law

The illuminance E_v at a point on a surface is inversely proportional to the square of the distance between the point and the source. Note that the variable r refers to the distance here.

$$E_v = \frac{I_v}{r^2} \tag{6.7}$$

6.3.2 Cosine Law

If the normal to an illuminated surface is at an angle θ to the direction of the incident light, the illuminance is proportional to the cosine of θ.

$$E_v = \frac{I_v}{r^2} \cdot \cos\theta \tag{6.8}$$

6.4 Exercises

1. Calculate the solid angle (ω) subtended at the center of a sphere with a diameter of $1\,m$, by an area of $2.5\,m^2$ on the surface of the sphere.
2. Calculate the illumination on a horizontal surface located $2\,m$ directly below a point source of light with the intensity of $200\,cd$.
3. A point light source with the intensity of $200\,cd$ is positioned at a distance of $2\,m$ from a horizontal surface. Calculate the illumination on that surface for a point that is located $1\,m$ away.

6.5 Further Reading

- Freeman MH, Hull CC. Optics. 11th Edition. Butterworth Heinemann. 2003.
- Lahiri, A. Basic Optics: Principles and Concepts., Elsevier Science. 2016.
- Tunnacliffe AH. Introduction to visual optics. London: Association of british dispensing opticians; 1993.
- Tunnacliffe AH., Hirst, JG, Optics. Association of British Dispensing Opticians. London; 1996.

Reference

1. Freeman MH, Hull CC. Optics. 11th ed. Butterworth Heinemann;2003.

7

Testing Visual Functions

In the following chapter, I will outline the most important concepts that are related to the measurement of important visual functions, such as visual acuity and contrast sensitivity. I will also introduce some relevant perceptual laws and units that are key to understand the measurement of visual functions.

7.1 Visual Acuity

The measurement of visual acuity is part of almost every eye examination. The goal is to measure the resolution limit of the eye/s for particular visual stimuli, also called optotypes (typically, letters or symbols). The resolution limit is expressed as the minimum angle of resolution (MAR) subtended by an optotype or a feature of the optotype. In general, the patient is asked to identify the letter or a row of letters. The size of the letters in the row is progressively decreased until the resolution limit is reached.

G. Schmidtmann, *Clinical Vision Science*,
https://doi.org/10.1007/978-3-031-83321-2_7

7.1.1 Visual Angle

In optometric practice and vision science, the image size is more informative than the physical size of the object. The image size is described by its visual angle θ subtended at the eye in degrees, or minutes/seconds of arc (see Sect. 1.2). Figure 7.1 shows the visual angle θ subtended by an object O with the height h at a viewing distance x. I refers to the image projected on the retina.

The visual angle θ for the scenario shown in Fig. 7.1 can be calculated according to the following equation.

$$\theta = \tan^{-1}\left(\frac{h}{x}\right) \tag{7.1}$$

In optometric practice, we test acuity for specially designed optotypes often presented on test charts. Figure 7.2 shows two common types of optotypes used in practice, the Tumbling E (top) and the Landolt C (bottom). Test charts are often standardized for a viewing distance of $6m$ (e.g., United Kingdom, Germany), or $20ft$ (e.g., USA). For this viewing distance, the design of the symbols leads to a visual angle

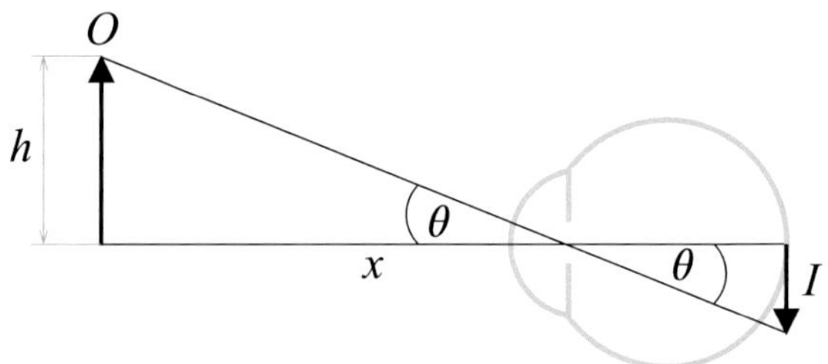

Fig. 7.1 Illustration of the visual angle θ subtended by the object O with the height h at a distance x. I refers to the image projected on the retina

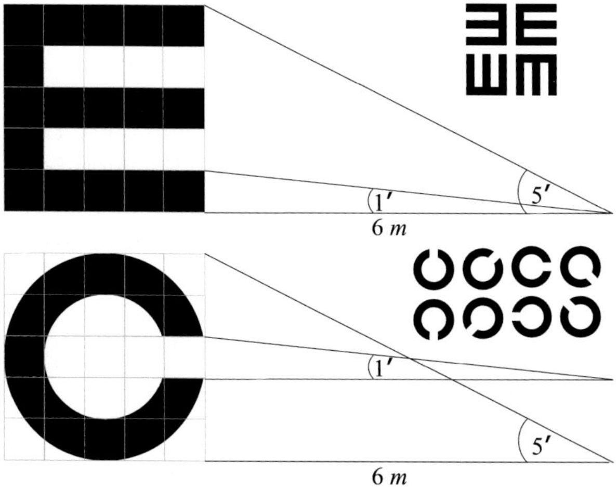

Fig. 7.2 The figure shows two common types of optotypes used in practice, the Tumbling E (top panel) and the Landolt C (bottom panel). The icons in the top right of each panel show the possible directions that the observer has to identify

subtended by the whole optotype of $5'$, and the discrete feature of resolution of $5'/5 = 1'$ (gap, or stroke width).[1]

The visual acuity V_a can be calculated according to the following equation.

$$V_a = \frac{d'}{d} \tag{7.2}$$

V_a: Visual acuity

d': Standard viewing distance (Metric: $6m$, or Imperial: $20\,ft$)

d: Distance at which the optotype subtends $5'$ (each element or gap subtends $1'$)

[1] Note that angles can be expressed in degrees or minutes and seconds of arc (arc min, arc sec, see Sect. 1.2.3).

7.1.2 Units of Visual Acuity and Conversions

The visual acuity can be expressed in various units. Different countries have adopted different units. The most common units and the conversion between them is summarized below. The minimum angle of resolution (MAR) is defined in arc minutes [′].

7.1.2.1 *log*MAR

$$logMAR = log_{10}MAR \tag{7.3}$$

7.1.2.2 Snellen Notation

Another very common unit is the Snellen notation or fraction. S_n be the numerator and S_d the denominator of the Snellen fraction. In the UK, S_d is typically set to 6, which refers to the distance between patient and test chart measured in m. Note that you can set S_d to any other distance, e.g., $4m$ [1].

*log*MAR can then be calculated according to:

$$logMAR = \log_{10}\left(\frac{S_n}{S_d}\right) \tag{7.4}$$

According to the calculation rules for logarithms, this equation can be rewritten as:

$$logMAR = \log_{10} S_n - \log_{10} S_d \tag{7.5}$$

7.1.2.3 Minimum Angle of Resolution (MAR)

The minimum angle of resolution (MAR) can then simply be calculated according to:

$$\text{MAR} = 10^{log\text{MAR}} \tag{7.6}$$

7.1.2.4 Decimal

Decimal *Dec* is defined as:

$$Dec = \frac{1}{\text{MAR}} \tag{7.7}$$

7.1.2.5 VAR

$$\text{VAR} = 100 - (50 \cdot log_{10}\text{MAR}) \tag{7.8}$$

7.1.3 Distance Vision

Tables 7.1 and 7.2 summarize common visual acuity units and their conversions for distance and near vision, respectively.

7.2 Contrast Measures

Another important clinical test of visual function is the patient's sensitivity to faint stimuli, i.e., the sensitivity to low-contrast stimuli or contrast sensitivity. The contrast is a measure of the difference in luminance between an object and its background. There are many different contrast measures. The most relevant ones are defined in the following sections.

Table 7.1 Visual acuity scales conversion table

MAR	*log*MAR	VAR	Snellen (Metric)	Snellen (Imperial)	Decimal
0.50	–0.30	115	6/3	20/10	2.00
0.63	–0.20	110	6/3.8	20/12.5	1.60
0.80	–0.10	105	6/4.8	20/16	1.25
1.00	0.00	100	6/6	20/20	1.00
1.25	0.10	95	6/7.5	20/25	0.80
1.60	0.20	90	6/9.5	20/32	0.63
2.00	0.30	85	6/12	20/40	0.50
2.50	0.40	80	6/15	20/50	0.40
3.20	0.50	75	6/19	20/63	0.32
4.00	0.60	70	6/24	20/80	0.25
5.00	0.70	65	6/30	20/100	0.20
6.30	0.80	60	6/38	20/125	0.16
8.00	0.90	55	6/48	20/160	0.125
10	1.00	50	6/60	20/200	0.10
20	1.30	35	6/120	20/400	0.05
40	1.60	20	6/240	20/800	0.025
100	2.00	0	6/600	20/2000	0.01

7.2.1 Weber Contrast

The Weber contrast is C_W is particularly useful to use when dealing with isolated features against a larger background (e.g., optotypes on test charts).

$$C_W = \frac{L - L_b}{L_b} \tag{7.9}$$

L: Luminance of target

L_b: Luminance of background

Table 7.2 Near visual acuity scales conversion table

*log*MAR	N-scale	M-units	Equivalent Snellen (Metric)	Equivalent Snellen (Imperial)
−0.10	2.50	0.32	6/5	20/16
0.00	3	0.40	6/6	20/20
0.10	4	0.50	6/7.5	20/25
0.20	5	0.60	6/9	20/30
0.30	6	0.75	6/12	20/40
0.40	8	1.0	6/15	20/50
0.50	10	1.2	6/18	20/60
0.60	12	1.6	6/24	20/80
0.70	16	2.0	6/30	20/100
0.80	20	2.5	6/36	20/125
0.90	25	3.2	6/48	20/160
1.00	32	4.0	6/60	20/200
1.10	40	5.0	6/75	20/250

7.2.2 Michelson Contrast

The Michelson contrast is useful for repeating patterns, such as periodic sine wave or square wave gratings (e.g., Functional Acuity Contrast Test, FACT [2]).

$$C_M = \frac{L_{max} - L_{min}}{L_{max} + L_{min}} \tag{7.10}$$

L_{max}: Maximum luminance

L_{min}: Minimum luminance

7.2.3 Root Mean Square (RMS) Contrast

The root mean square or RMS contrast is typically employed for more complex patterns, such as natural images [3, 4].

$$C_i = \frac{(L_i - L)}{L} = \frac{\Delta L_i}{L} \tag{7.11}$$

where L_i is the luminance of the i_{th} pixel and L is the average lumininance.

$$C_{\mathrm{RMS}} = \left(n^{-1} \sum_{i=0}^{n} C_i^2\right)^{0.5} \tag{7.12}$$

C_{RMS}: Root mean square contrast

7.3 Contrast Sensitivity

The contrast sensitivity is a measure of the sensitivity to stimuli of varying contrast. These stimuli can be letters (e.g., Pelli-Robson chart [5]), or sinusoidal gratings (e.g., CSV-1000 chart, Vector Vision®).

7.3.1 Sinusoidal Gratings

Sinusoidal gratings are periodic patterns of sinusoidal modulations of the luminance. Figure 7.3 shows examples of sinusoidal gratings with different spatial frequencies.

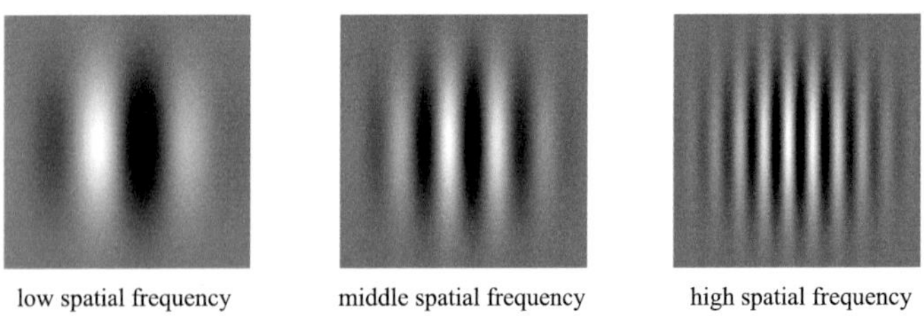

Fig. 7.3 The figure shows examples of sinusoidal gratings with low, middle and high spatial frequencies

7.3.1.1 Spatial Frequency

Like the sinusoidal function covered in Sect. 1.4.1, a sinusoidal grating is defined by its amplitude, frequency, and phase. The amplitude modulates the maximum and minimum luminance (i.e., contrast). The frequency changes the occurence of light and dark bands (Fig. 7.3). In the context of sinusoidal gratings, the frequency is called spatial frequency, which is measured in cycles per degree (also often abbreviated as cpd, or c/deg, etc.). The phase changes the position of light and dark bands (see Fig. 1.5). In addition, it is also possible to change the overall orientation of the grating; e.g., to create a grating that is tilted, where all the bars are diagonal instead of vertical as the bars depicted in Fig. 7.3.

7.3.2 The Contrast Sensitivity Function

The contrast sensitivity function (CSF) shows the contrast sensitivity (1/contrast detection threshold) for sinusoidal

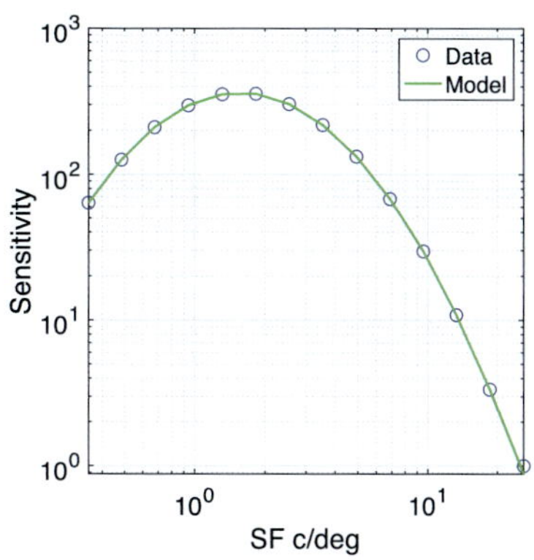

Fig. 7.4 The figure shows an illustration of a contrast sensitivity function. Contrast sensitivity is plotted as a function of spatial frequency (SF) measured in cycles per degree of visual angle [c/deg]

gratings with different spatial frequencies. An example is shown in Fig. 7.4.

7.4 Perceptual Laws

7.4.1 Weber's Law

The ability to perceive a difference between two stimuli of varying intensity is referred to as discriminability. The discriminability between two near stimuli, S and $S + \Delta S$ that differ by the increment ΔS (just noticeable difference), can be measured at various stimulus intensities. When Ernst Heinrich Weber (1795–1878) measured ΔS, he realized that it was proportional to the magnitude of the baseline stimulus; a relationship that is now known as "Weber's law" [6].

$$\Delta S = S \cdot k \tag{7.13}$$

or

$$\frac{\Delta S}{S} = k \tag{7.14}$$

where k is a constant referred to as "Weber fraction".

ΔS: Just Noticable Difference

S: Stimulus intensity

k: Weber fraction

7.4.2 Fechner's Law

Gustav Fechner (1801–1887) subsequently revised Weber's law to relate the intensity S (i.e., magnitude) of a stimulus and the perceived magnitude P [7].

$$P = k \cdot \log S \tag{7.15}$$

P: Perceived magnitude

S: Stimulus intensity

k: Weber fraction

7.4.3 Steven's Power Law

Stanley Smith Stevens (1906–1973) established the following relationship between the perceived magnitude P evoked by a stimulus and the stimulus intensity [8].

$$P = \alpha \cdot S^n \tag{7.16}$$

P: Perceived magnitude

S: Stimulus intensity

α: scaling factor ($\alpha = 1$ linear; $\alpha < 1$ compressive; $\alpha > 1$ expansive)

n: power exponent

7.5 Exercises

1. A Tumbling E is presented at a distance of $6m$. A patient achieves a visual acuity of $-0.1 log$MAR.
   a. What is the size of a single stroke (stroke width, S_w) of the Tumbling E?
   b. What is the overall size S of the Tumbling E in mm?

2. Convert the minimum angle of resolution MAR $= 0.63'$ into a Snellen fraction, assuming a viewing distance of $6m$.

7.6 Further Reading

- Bruce V, Green PR, Georgeson MA. Visual perception: Physiology, psychology, & ecology. Psychology Press; 2003.
- Prins N, Kingdom FAA. Psychophysics: a practical introduction. Academic Press; 2016.
- Snowden R, Thompson P, Troscianko T. Basic vision: an introduction to visual perception. Oxford University Press; 2012.
- Goldstein EB. Sensation and perception. Cengage Learning; 2009.

References

1. Bailey IL, Lovie JE. New design principles for visual acuity letter charts. Optomet Vis Sci. 1976;53(11):740–5.
2. Ginsburg AP. Next generation contrast sensitivity testing. Function Assess Low Vis. 1996;77–88.
3. Rovamo J, Franssila R, Näsänen R. Contrast sensitivity as a function of spatial frequency, viewing distance and eccentricity with and without spatial noise. Vis Res. 1992;32(4):631–7.
4. Legge GE, Kersten D, Burgess AE. Contrast discrimination in noise. JOSA A. 1987;4(2):391–404.
5. Pelli DG, Robson JG, Wilkins AJ. The design of a new letter chart for measuring contrast sensitivity. Clin Vis Sci. 1988;2:187–99.
6. Weber EH. De pulsu, resorptione, auditu et tactu: annotationes anatomicae et physiologicae, auctore. prostat apud CF Koehler; 1834.

7. Fechner GT, Howes DH, Boring EG. Elements of psychophysics. New York: Holt, Rinehart and Winston; 1966.
8. Stevens SS. On the psychophysical law. Psychol Rev. 1957;64(3):153–81.

8

Clinical Procedures

The following chapter contains short descriptions and custom-made flow charts to simplify the necessary steps to establish a patient's prescription, observe the eye via slit lamp biomicroscopy, and measure the radii of the cornea using a keratometer.

8.1 Basics

Knowing the patient's visual acuity without correction allows us to estimate the amount of spherical ametropia. Table 8.1 shows these estimations.

G. Schmidtmann, *Clinical Vision Science*,
https://doi.org/10.1007/978-3-031-83321-2_8

Table 8.1 Blur estimation table

Visual acuity	Sphere [DS]	Cylinder [DC]
6/5	0–0.25	0.25
6/6	0.25	0.50
6/9	0.50	1.00
6/12	0.75	1.50
6/18	1.00	2.00
6/24	1.25	2.50
6/36	1.75	3.50
6/60	2.50	5.00
3/36	3.00	6.00
3/60	4.00	8.00
1/24	4.50	9.00
1/36	5.75	11.50
1/60	7.50	15.00

8.2 Retinoscopy

8.2.1 Working Distance Lens

Before you start with retinoscopy, it is essential to measure the working distance and to calculate the working distance lens that is required. Table 8.2 shows some common work distances and the corresponding lenses.

Table 8.2 Working distance lens

Working distance [cm]	Lens sphere [DS]
20	+5.00
~22	+4.50
25	+4.00
33	+3.00
40	+2.50
50	+2.00
~66.7	+1.50

8.2.2 Retinoscopy–Procedure

Retinoscopy (static) is a method to objectively determine the sphero-cylindrical refractive error and the extent of a regular (or irregular) astigmatism. A streak of light is shone into the eye and the examiner interprets the retinal reflex. There are three main directions of the retinal reflex–I neutral, II with movement and III against movement; these are illustrated in Fig. 8.1.

Remember
- With movement: hyperopia–add postive lens
- Against movement: myopia–add minus lens
- Neutral: emmetrope.

Remember to judge these movements in various directions (see Fig. 8.2).

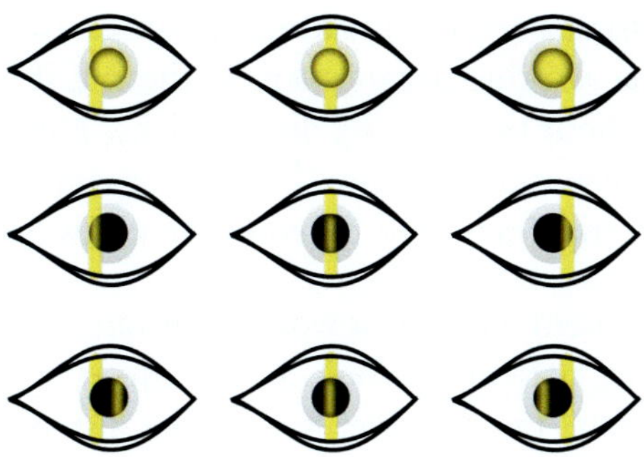

Fig. 8.1 The figures shows a streak of light which moves from left to right. Pupil reflex direction: neutral (top), with movement (middle) and against movement (bottom)

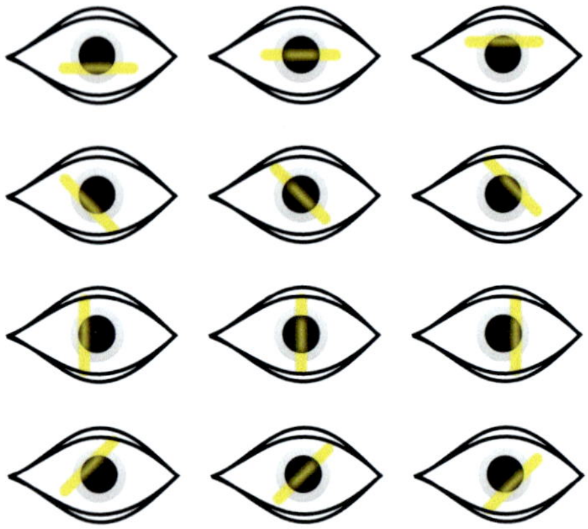

Fig. 8.2 The figures shows a streak of light at various directions

The retinoscopy procedure described below assumes that you have measured the inter-pupillary distance (PD) and have fit the trial frame. Please make sure that you dim the room illumination. We further assume that you perform retinoscopy with a working distance lens. Table 8.2 shows working distance lenses for various distances. Remember to subtract the working distance lens at the end if you decide to work without the working distance lens. The easiest way is to add the working distance lens as a separate lens in the back of the trial frame and to remove it afterwards.

1. Set up patient and adjust working distance.
2. Ask your patient to look at the green panel of the Duochrome test (see Fig. 8.3) in the distance to minimize (control) accommodation.

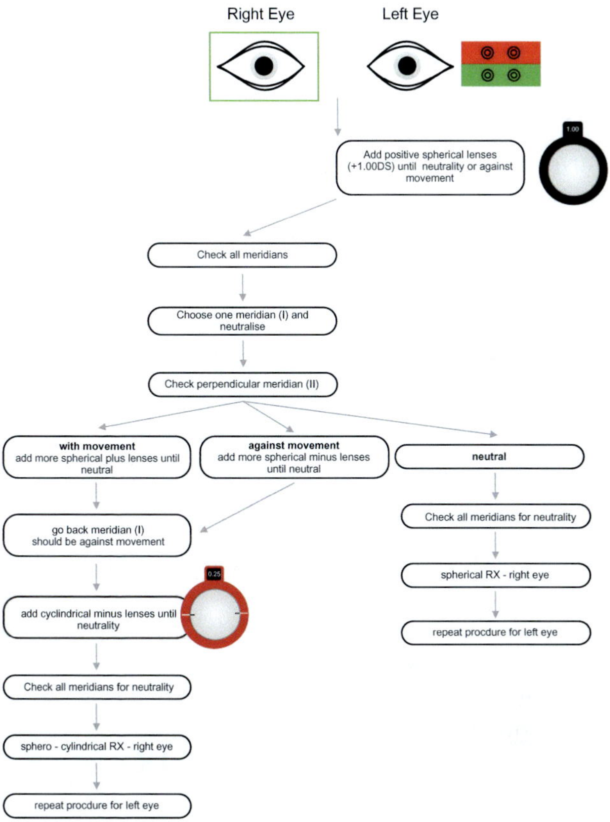

Fig. 8.3 The flow chart shows the retinoscopy procedure for the right eye

3. Shine light into to be tested eye and observe reflex to see that you are on axis.
4. Shine light into the left eye.
   - If you observe with movement, then add plus lenses in +1.00 DS steps until you observe neutrality or against movement.

5. Shine light into the right eye and check the movement in all meridians (see Fig. 8.2).
6. Choose one meridian and neutralize the meridian by adding the appropriate spherical lenses (see Fig. 8.1).
7. Turn the retinoscope to the perpendicular meridian and check the reflex.
   - If this meridian is neutral, you have corrected a spherical refractive error.
   - If you observe a with movement, add more spherical plus lenses until it is neutralized.
   - Go back to the original meridian.
   - It will now show an against movement.
   - Use cylindrical minus lenses with the axis in this meridian to achieve neutrality.
8. Add –0.50 DC with the axis in line with the streak.
   - If you observe with movement, replace –0.50 DC with –0.25 DC.
   - If you observe against movement, add –0.50 DC until you observe with movement.
   - Finally, reduce the cylinder by 0.25 DC.
9. Check all meridians for neutrality.

8.3 Subjective Refraction

In the following section, we will cover subjective measurements of the sphero-cylindrical refractive error and the extent of a regular (or irregular) astigmatism.

Table 8.3 Sphere refinement

Visual acuity	Lens sphere [DS]
$\leq$ 6/12	±0.25
6/18–6/60	±0.50
$\geq$ 6/60	±1.00

8.3.1 Best Vision Sphere

First, we have to ensure to establish the best vision sphere, which is the maximum positive spherical plus lens, or the minimum minus spherical lens, to achieve the highest possible visual acuity. This ensures that the circle of least confusion is on the retina (see Sect. 3.7).

Note that it is important to use a suitable sphere lens, depending on the patient's visual acuity (see Table 8.3).

Remember

- The best vision sphere is the spherical lens that creates a mixed astigmatism, i.e., the circle of least confusion is on the retina.
- The best vision sphere is the maximum positive spherical plus lens, or the minimum minus spherical lens to achieve the highest possible visual acuity.

The following two flow charts demonstrate the procedure for the determination of the best vision sphere for hyperopia and myopia (Figs. 8.4 and 8.5).

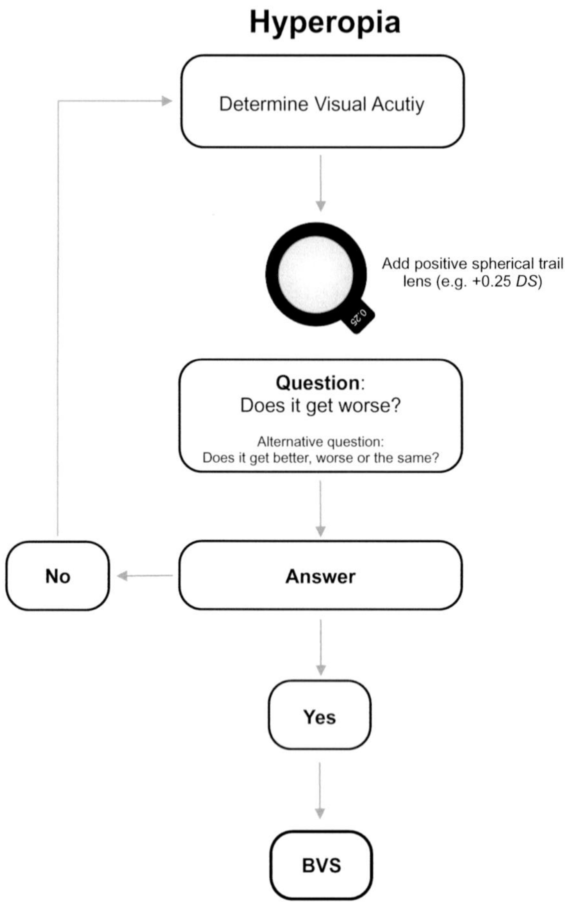

Fig. 8.4 Flow Chart for the determination of the best vision sphere for hyperopia

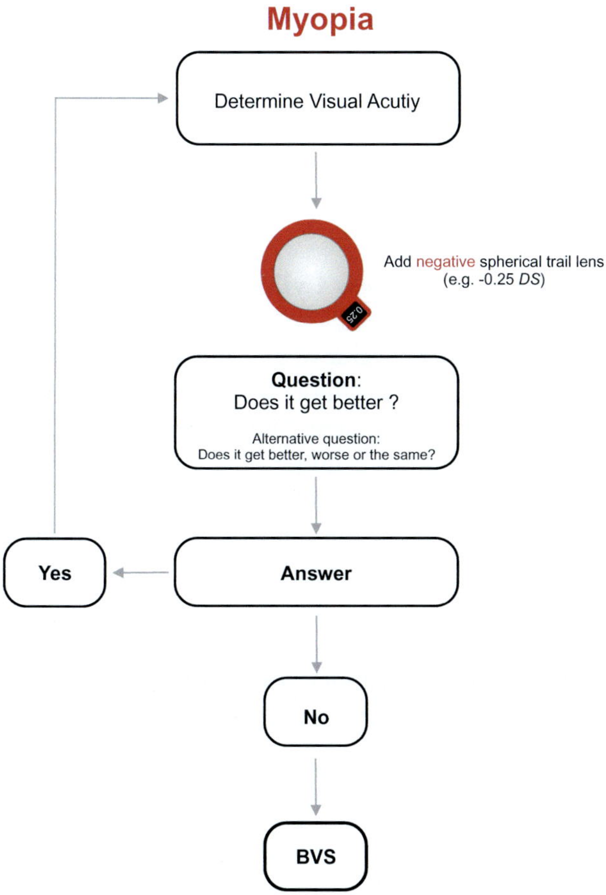

Fig. 8.5 Flow Chart for the determination of the best vision sphere for myopia

8.3.2 Jackson Cross Cylinder

In the following section, we will cover the Jackson cross cylinder method, which is a common method to measure and refine the cylinder power and axis during refraction using a Jackson cross cylinder.

8.3.2.1 Power of Cross Cylinder

A cross cylinder with a value of ± C is composed of a sphere with a power of C and a cylinder with a power of 2 C with an opposite sign than the sphere. The axis of the cross cylinder is the axis of the minus cylinder (Fig. 8.6). Common cross cylinder powers are ±0.12, ±0.25, ±0.50, and ±1.00. Similar to the power of the spherical lens used in the best vision sphere routine, the power of the cross cylinder used is dependent on the visual acuity of the patient (see Table 8.4). Figures 8.7 and 8.8 illustrate the procedures to determine the cylinder axis and cylinder power, respectively.

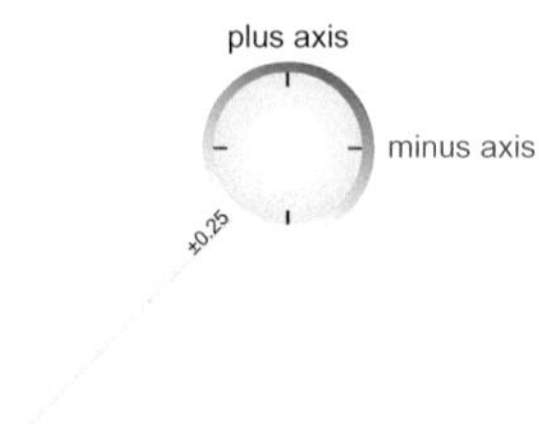

Fig. 8.6 Jackson cross cylinder

Table 8.4 Sphere refinement

Visual acuity	Cross cylinder power [D]
≤ 6/12	±0.25
6/18–6/60	±0.50
≥ 6/60	±1.00

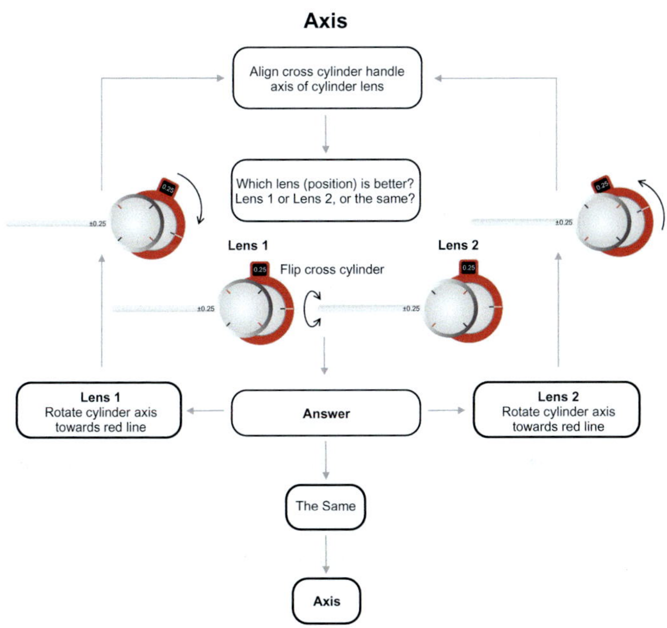

Fig. 8.7 Flowchart for the determination of the cylinder axis

Remember

- For every –0.50 DC increase in cylinder you should add a sphere of +0.25 DS
- For every +0.50 DC increase in cylinder you should add a sphere of –0.25 DS.

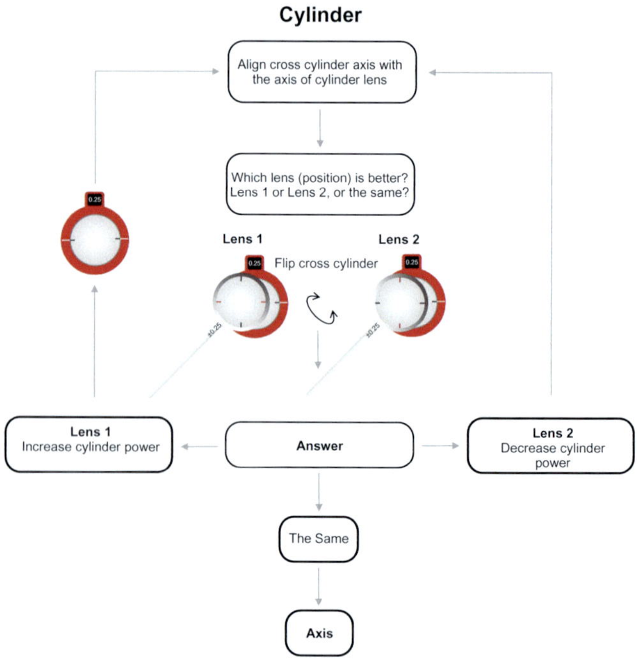

Fig. 8.8 Flowchart for the determination of the cylinder power

8.4 Slit Lamp Biomicroscopy

Optically, the slit lamp is a microscope with an illumination system. The observation system (microscope) and the illumination system rotate around a common axis of rotation (Fig. 8.9).

8.4.1 Focusing of the Eyepieces

It is very important to focus the eyepieces (oculars) before any slit lamp examination or the usage of any other optical instrument (e.g., keratometer, focimeter, etc.). There are two

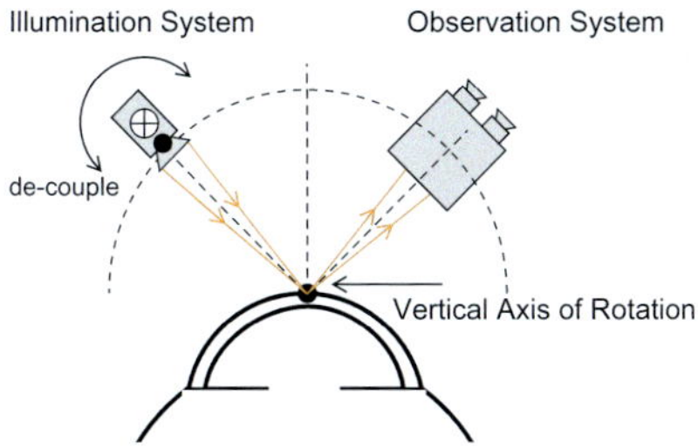

Fig. 8.9 Slit lamp general principle

ways to focus the eyepieces of a slit lamp, depending on whether there is a focusing rod available or not.

8.4.1.1 With Focusing Rod

- Rotate the microscope into a straight position
- Place the focusing rod into the designated hole at the pivot point (axis of rotation)
- Rotate the focusing rod so that the flat side is facing the microscope
- Adjust the slit width to about 1 *mm* with medium/high intensity
- Swing the illumination system and make sure the slit does not move
- It is decoupled or not calibrated if the slit moves
- Focus the eyepieces (see below).

8.4.1.2 Without Focusing Rod

- Rotate the microscope into a straight position

- Adjust the slit width to about 1 *mm* with medium/high intensity and place it at the flat part between your patient's eyebrows
- Alternatively, you can place a sheet of paper at the chin and forehead rest at the position where the forehead would be located
- Move the slit lamp with the joystick so that the pivot point (axis of rotation; focusing rod hole) is roughly at the same plane as the forehead or sheet of paper
- Swing the illumination system and find the position where the slit does not move
- Focus the eyepieces (see below).

Focusing the Eyepieces

- Rotate the eyepieces towards positive/plus (usually counter-clockwise)
- Monocularly turn the eyepieces towards negative/minus until the slit is focused
- Double-check binocularly.

8.4.2 Slit Lamp Illumination Techniques

8.4.2.1 Diffuse Illumination

See Fig. 8.10

Applications

- Diffuse illumination is ideal to get a general overview of the external eye, the eyelids and lid margins, eyelashes, plica, caruncle, sclera and cornea, etc.
- It can also be applied for the assessment of contact lens fit

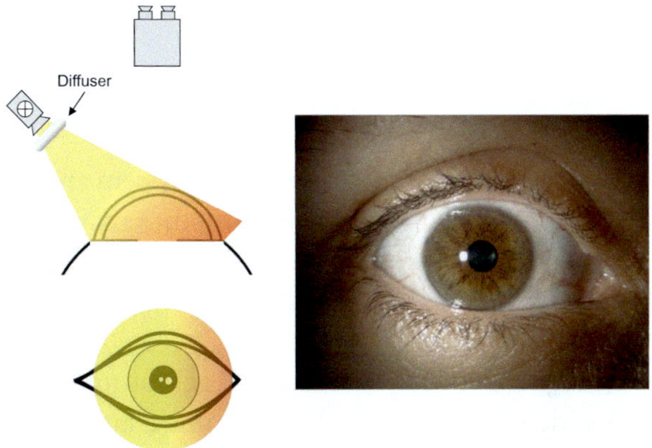

Fig. 8.10 Diffuse illumination, Photo: Gunnar Schmidtmann

Procedure

- Increase the slit width (wide bream) and the light intensity (medium to high illumination)
- Use a diffuser and investigate the external structures with a low to medium magnification
- This technique is not very useful if you want to investigate detailed structures.

8.4.2.2 Direct Illumination

Applications

- This technique is suitable for the assessment of cataracts, scars, nerves, blood vessels, etc.
- It can also be applied for the determination of the axis of toric contact lenses

Procedure

- Place the illumination system at an angle of about 40° to 50°
- The light beam from the illumination system and microscope are focused on the ocular structure that you want to investigate
- Move the entire system towards the structure you want to investigate
- Remember the focus plane is at the axis of rotation
- Use a wide beam (2–3 *mm*) to examine a large area.

8.4.2.3 Parallelepiped

Applications

- The parallelepiped is useful to examine corneal structures and defects, such as scars and foreign bodies

Procedure

- Use a narrow slit of about 1–3 *mm*, medium to high intensity
- Use medium to high magnification
- Illuminate a rectangular section of the cornea
- The microscope should be positioned in front of patient's eye/cornea
- Place the illumination system at an angle of about 45°
- Variable magnification, medium to high.

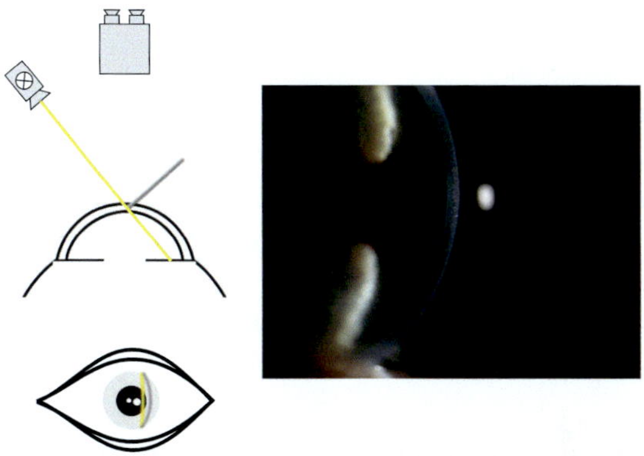

Fig. 8.11 Direct illumination/Optic section of the cornea, Photo: Mahesh R. Joshi

8.4.2.4 Optic Section

See Fig. 8.11.

Applications

- The optic section is useful to examine corneal defects in great detail

Procedure

- An optic section is a very thin parallelepiped (narrowest possible slit; $<1\,mm$), creating a very thin slice of the cornea
- Adjust the axes of the illumination system and microscope so that they intersect in the location of the medium to be examined
- Place the illumination system at an angle of about 45°
- Use a the narrowest slit to examine the depth of foreign bodies
- Use maximum magnification.

8.4.2.5 Conical Section

Applications

- To examine the transparency of the anterior chamber
- To detect floating cells and flare seen in e.g., anterior uveitis (Tyndall effect)

Procedure

- A conical beam is created by reducing the height of a parallelepiped (1–3 *mm*) to produce a small circular or square spot of light
- Place the illumination system temporally at an angle of about 45° to 60° and direct it towards the pupil
- The microscope should be positioned in front of the patient's eye/cornea in a straight position
- Use medium to high magnification (16–25x) and high intensity
- Focus the beam between cornea and anterior lens surface and dark zone between cornea and anterior lens observed
- The principle is the same as that of a beam of sunlight streaming through a room, illuminating airborne dust particles.

8.4.2.6 Sclerotic Scatter

See Fig. 8.12.

Application

- The Sclerotic scatter technique is ideal to observe corneal opacities, e.g., corneal oedema

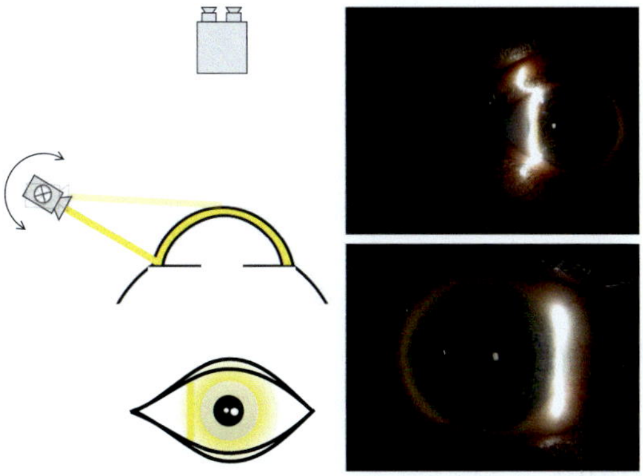

Fig. 8.12 Slerotic scatter, Photos: Mahesh R. Joshi & Joao Alhada Lourenco

Procedure

- Sclerotic scatter is an illumination technique that utilizes the phenomenon of total internal reflection (see Sect. 2.2.4)
- To apply the sclerotic scatter technique use a bright and narrow slit of approximately 1 *mm* and place the slit on the limbus region (preferably temporal)
- Move the illumination unit to an angle of about 40° to 60° until the entire limbus starts to glow
- Use a low or no magnification and search the cornea for opacities
- Uncouple the illumination unit for direct focal illumination.

8.4.2.7 Indirect Illumination

See Fig. 8.13.

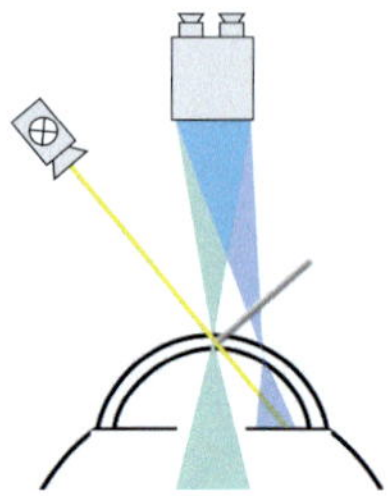

Fig. 8.13 Indirect illumination

Applications

- Indirect illumination is useful to examine objects in direct vicinity of corneal areas of reduced transparency, e.g., corneal scars, deposits, epithelial and stromal anomalities

Procedure

- The set up is identical to the direct illumination (cyan in Fig. 8.13)
- Examine the ocular structures which are indirectly illuminated (blue in Fig. 8.13)
- Focus on the structure of interest
- Use a narrow to medium slit width and a medium magnification (12x).

8.4.2.8 Retro Illumination

See Fig. 8.14.

Applications

- Retro-illuminated structures appear darker

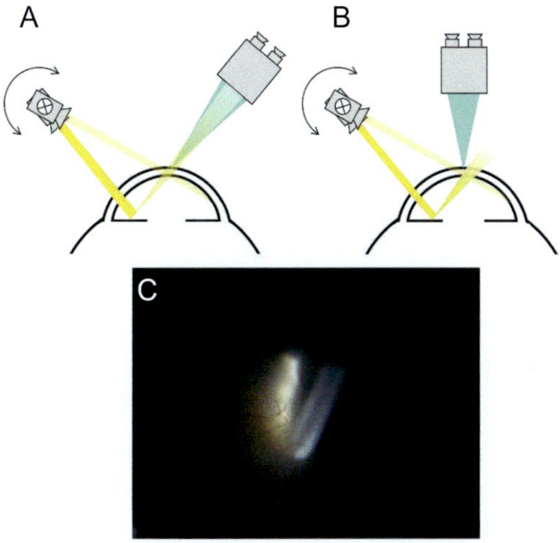

Fig. 8.14 (**A**) direct retro illumination, (**B**) indirect retro illumination, (**C**) retro illuminated blood vessels of the peripheral cornea, Photo: Joao Alhada Lourenco

- It is useful to examine neovascularizations of the cornea, microcysts and infiltrates
- Retro illumination can also be used to examine the crystalline lens using the retina as the reflection plane (e.g., posterior subcapsular cataract)

Procedure

- The light is reflected from a surface (usually the iris) and the structure of interest is illuminated from behind
- Direct and indirect observations are possible, depending on the position of the microscope (see Fig. 8.14)
- Use a slit with of 1–4 *mm*, medium illumination and variable magnification.

8.4.2.9 Specular Reflection

Applications

- This technique is mainly used to investigate the corneal endothelium (second Purkinje image)

Procedure

- Specular reflection is a subtype of direct illumination
- It uses the principles of relection (see Sect. 2.3)
- Set the slit lamp so that the illumination system and microscope are opposite to each other (see Fig. 8.15)
- The angle of incidence and angle of reflection should be around 25° each
- Use a narrow–medium slit width and medium intensity
- Start with a low magnification
- Adjust the slit lamp so that the tear film is in focus (ask your patient to blink and you will see the particles moving in the tear film)
- Find the bright spot (reflection) and move it into the center of your field of view
- Increase the magnification and adjust centration

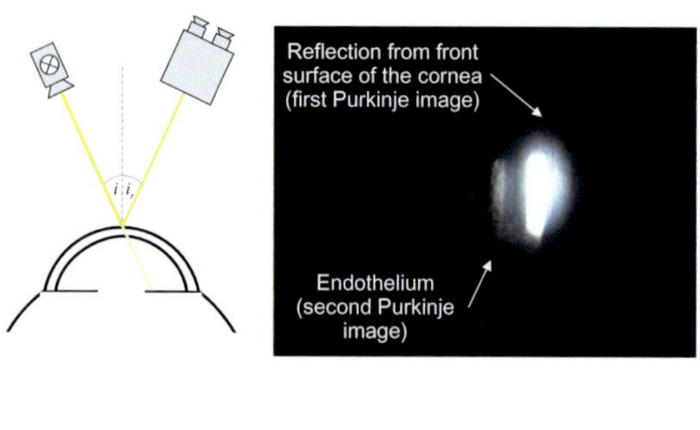

Fig. 8.15 Specular reflection/corneal endothelium, Photo: Joao Alhada Lourenco

- Continue this process until you reach maximum magnification
- The first Purkinje image is the bright reflection on the front surface of the cornea
- The slightly less bright (golden) image adjacent to the first Purkinje image is the back surface of the cornea (corneal endothelium, second Purkinje image)
- Gently move the slit lamp back and forth to focus the slit lamp on the corneal endothelium
- Increase the slit width to increase the section of the corneal endothelium
- The corneal endothelium resembles a mosaic-like pattern
- This technique requires steady hands.

8.4.2.10 van Herick's Technique

Applications

- The van Herick's technique [3] is a slit lamp technique that allows the estimation of the anterior chamber angle

Procedure

- Move the illumination system to an angle of precisely 60° temporal
- The microscope system should be positioned in front of patient's eye/cornea in a straight position
- Create an optic section of the cornea and move the slit adjacent to the temporal limbus on the sclera
- Use the narrowest slit available and increase the light intensitiy to maxium
- Move the optic section towards the limbus until the first optic section of the cornea will be visible

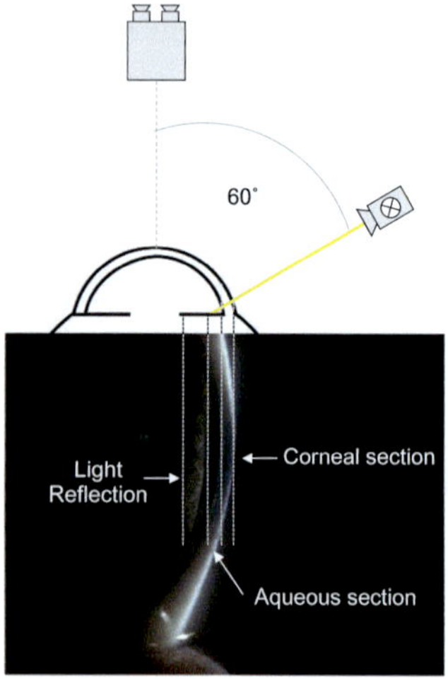

Fig. 8.16 van Herrick technique, Photo: Mahesh R. Joshi

Table 8.5 van Herick's grades

Ratio (Aqueous section/Corneal section)	Grade	Anterior chamber angle
< 1/4	Grade 1	Dangerously narrow/likely to close
1/3	Grade 2	Very narrow
1/2	Grade 3	Narrow
≥ 1/1	Grade 4	Wide open angle

- Estimate the ratio between aqueous and corneal section (see Fig. 8.16)
- Assess the van Herick Grade according to Table 8.5.

8.5 Keratometry

The measurement of the corneal topography, i.e., the corneal curvature or radii, is called keratometry. This procedure is essential for the fitting of contact lenses, but can also be used to assess the corneal refractive power and astigmatism and to investigate corneal abnormalities, for example keratoconus or keratoglobus. The optical instrument to measure the central corneal radii is the *keratometer* (also called Ophthalmometer). The keratometer projects two test images, so-called mire images, onto the cornea and its tear film, which acts as a convex mirror. The examiner adjusts the positions of the mire images by changing the angle of incidence and reflection until they coincide. A non-spherical (toric) cornea requires the measurement of the corneal radius in both meridians. There are various types of keratometer, but they can be subdivided into two main categories.

1. One-Position
2. Two-Position

Two-Position keratometers require a rotation of 90° to measure the corneal radius for each meridian. Keratometers typically provide the corneal radii (r_c) in *mm* and the corresponding refractive power (F_c), which are related according to the following equation:

$$r_C = \frac{337.5}{F_c} \tag{8.1}$$

$$F_c = \frac{337.5}{r_C} \tag{8.2}$$

F_c: Refractive Power of cornea

r_c: Corneal radius in *mm*

8.5.1 Keratometry–Procedure

8.5.1.1 One-Position (Bausch and Lomb Keratometer)

The illustration below shows examples of the mire images for a ®Bausch & Lomb keratometer. The procedures described below assume a toric, non-spherical cornea.

- Focus the eyepieces (see Sect. 8.4.1)
- Position the keratometer
- The mire images might appear at a random position and might be blurry
- Adjust the keratometer so that the mire images appear focused and in the middle of the field of view
- Note that the horizontal + and the vertical – signs are not aligned

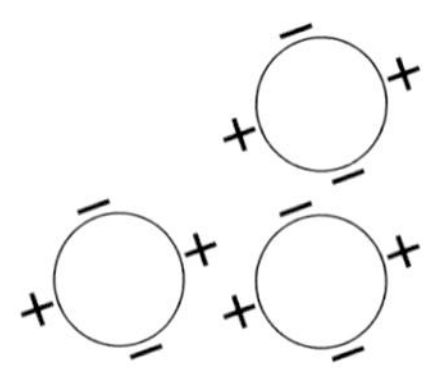

Horizontal Meridian

- Rotate the ®Bausch & Lomb keratometer to align the horizontal + and vertcial – signs

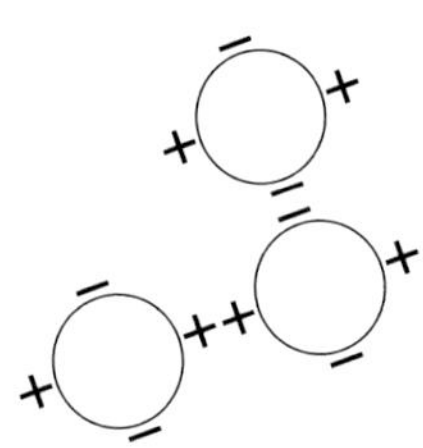

- Adjust the horizontal radius to align the horizontal + signs

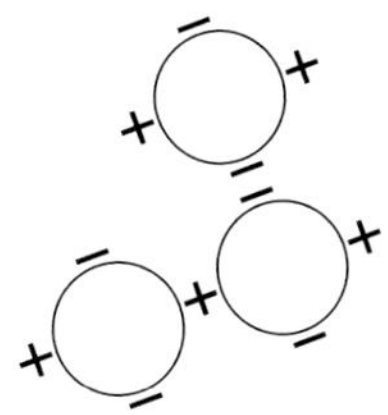

Vertical Meridian

- Adjust the vertical radius to align the vertical – signs
- Note that the One-Position keratometers do not require you to actively rotate the instrument to measure the vertical position

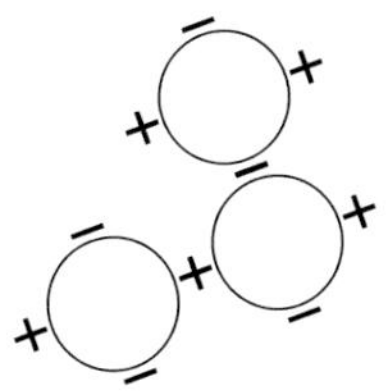

- Read off the radii and corresponding axes from the scale.

8.5.1.2 Two-Position Keratometer (®Zeiss and ®Javal-Schiotz)

The illustrations below show examples of the mire images for a ®Zeiss (left) and a ®Javal-Schiotz (right) keratometer. The procedures described below assume a toric, non-spherical cornea. Two-Position keratometers require the examiner to actively rotate the instrument to measure the horizontal and vertical meridians.

- Focus the eyepieces (see Sect. 8.4.1)
- Position the keratometer
- The mire images might appear at a random position and might be blurry

- Rotate the ®Zeiss or ®Javal-Schiotz keratometer into a horizontal position
- Adjust the keratometer so that the mire images appear focused and in the middle of the field of view
- Note that the mire images are not aligned (i.e., the two mire images do not coincide)

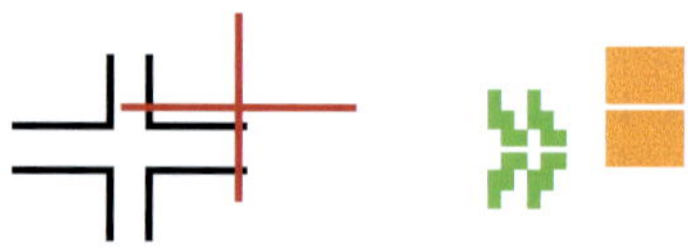

Horizontal Meridian

- Rotate the keratometer along the horizontal meridian (±40°) until the mire images are aligned (as shown in image below)

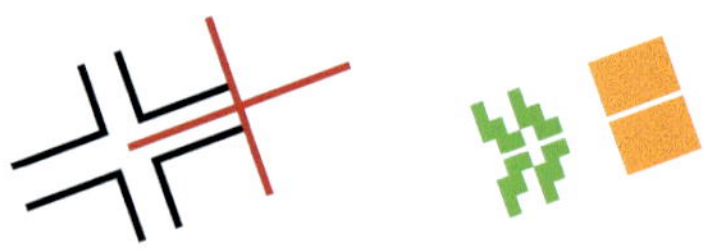

- Adjust the radius scale until the mire images are aligned, i.e., in conicidence
- Read off the radius and corresponding axis from the scale

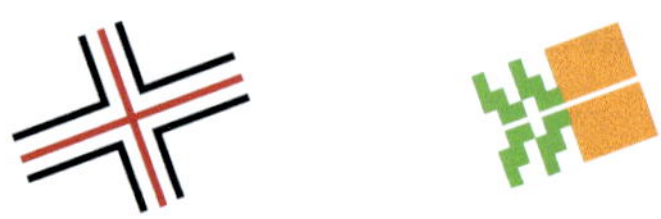

- Rotate the keratometer by 90°

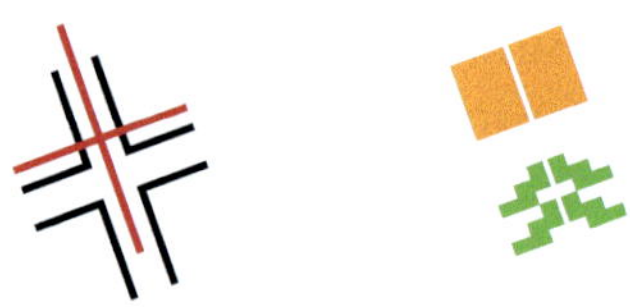

- Adjust the radius scale until the mire images are aligned, i.e., in conicidence
- Read off the radius and corresponding axis from the scale.

8.6 Further Reading

- Elliott DB. Clinical procedures in primary eye care. Elsevier Health Sciences; 2020 Jan 30.

Reference

1. van Herick W, Shaffer RN, Schwartz A. Estimation of width of angle of anterior chamber: incidence and significance of the narrow angle. Am J Ophthalmol. 1969;68(4):626–9.

9

Anatomy and Binocular Vision

Ocular anatomy and binocular vision are important and major subjects in the clinical vision sciences, and each topic could fill many volumes. In the following chapter, I will provide illustrations of important anatomical structures, such as the eye, the retina and the extraocular eye muscles, as well as schematics of the visual pathway, the pupil reflex pathway, the cranial nerves and many more. This chapter also seeks to illustrate some tests to assess common binocular vision problems.

9.1 Anatomy of the External Eye and Lacrimal System

The upper image of Fig. 9.1 shows some anatomical structures of the external eye (left eye), whereas the bottom image illustrates the key structures of the lacrimal system.

G. Schmidtmann, *Clinical Vision Science*,
https://doi.org/10.1007/978-3-031-83321-2_9

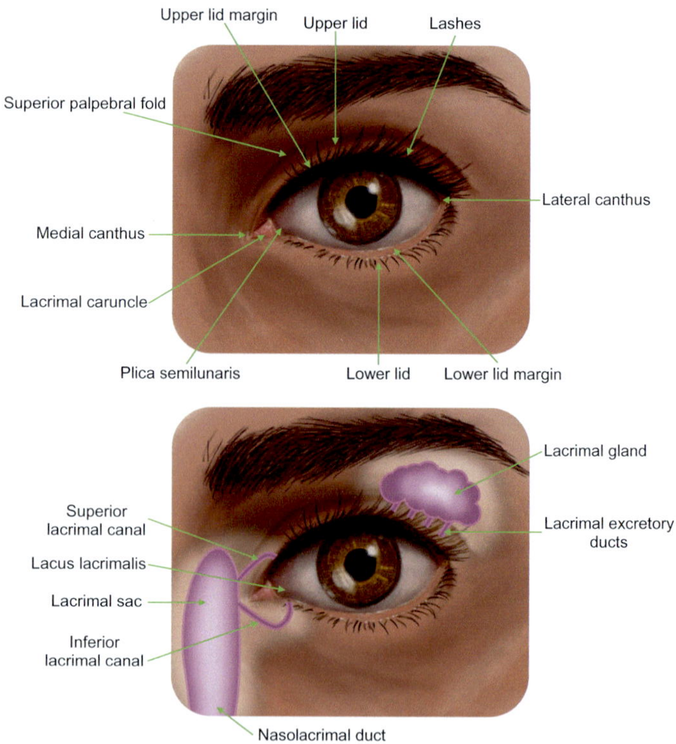

Fig. 9.1 The upper image shows an illustration of anatomical structures of the external human eye with various labels. The lower image shows the key structures of the lacrimal system. Illustration: Samantha Strong (https://samstrongvision.com)

The human lacrimal system is responsible for the production and drainage of tears, which help lubricate, nourish, and protect the eyes. It consists of the lacrimal glands, located temporally above each eye, which produce tears. The tears reach the eye via the lacrimal excretory ducts, and are spread across the surface of the eye when we blink. The tears then drain through the superior and inferior lacrimal canals into the lacrimal sac, eventually flowing into the nasolacrimal duct, which empties into the nasal cavity.[1] This system plays a crucial role in maintaining eye health by keeping the eye surface moist and flushing away irritants.

9.2 Anatomy of the Eye

Figure 9.2 shows an illustration of a cross-section of a human eye with labels for the most important anatomical structures.

Figure 9.3 shows a simplified schematic of the retina with labels for the layers and most important cell types.

9.2.1 Anatomy of the Retina

Figure 9.4 shows a photograph of a human retina (also called fundus) of a right eye taken with a fundus camera with labels indicating the most important structures.

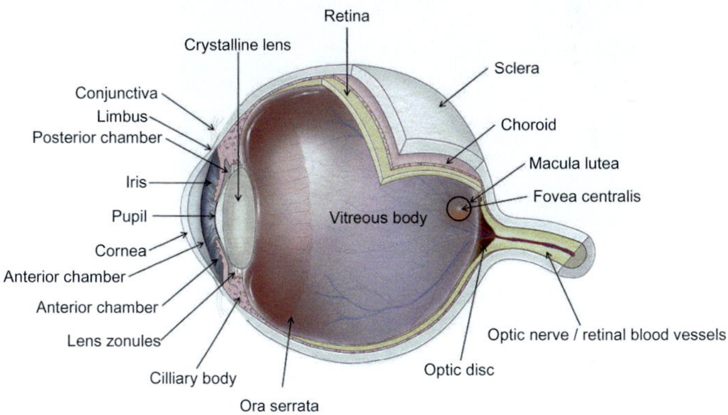

Fig. 9.2 The figure shows an illustration of the human eye with its various structures. Illustration: Sae Bom Ra

[1]Note that the nasal cavity is not shown in Fig. 9.1.

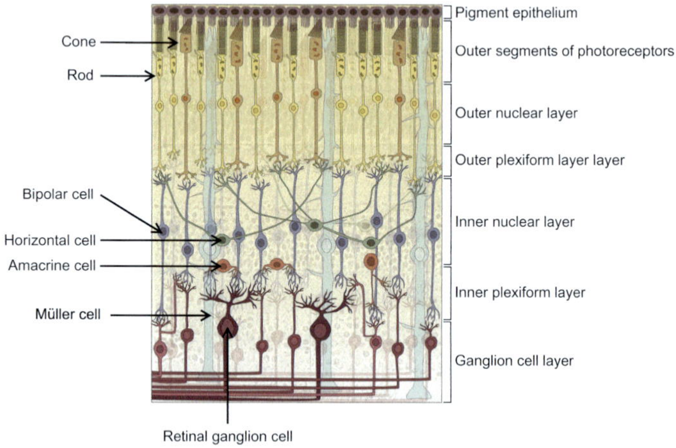

Fig. 9.3 The figure shows an illustration of a cross-section of a human retina with its various layers and types of cells. Illustration: Sae Bom Ra

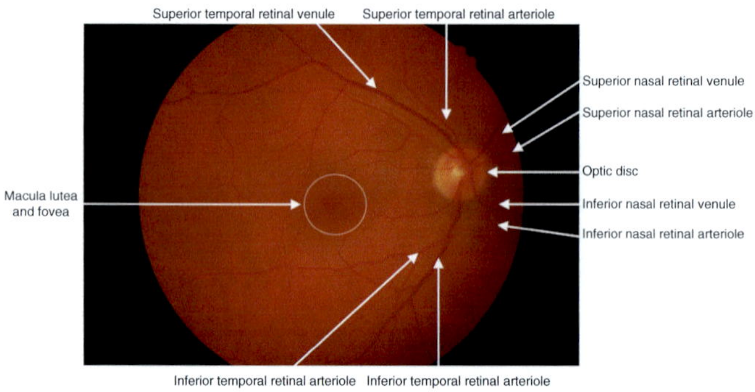

Fig. 9.4 The figure shows a fundus picture of the retina of a right eye with some important structures, arteries and veins. Photo: Gunnar Schmidtmann

9.3 The Visual Pathway

It is essential and clinically of upmost importance to understand the visual pathways in detail. Figure 9.5 shows an illustration of the visual pathway and common visual field defects and the associated location of injury/lesions.

The left visual field, illustrated as the light blue semi-circle in the upper part of the schematic, is projected onto the nasal retina of the left eye and the temporal retina of the right eye (dark blue/purple). The information from the nasal retina of the left eye is carried by the optic nerve (CN II) crosses over at the optic chiasm and forms the right optic tract,

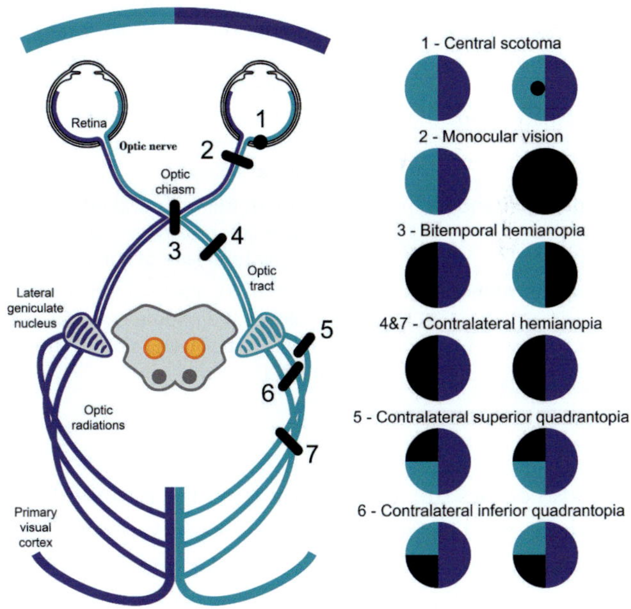

Fig. 9.5 The figure shows a schematic illustration of the visual pathway, prominent structures and their terminology and common visual field defects depending of the location of injury (1–7). Illustration: Samantha Strong (https://samstrongvision.com)

Table 9.1 Common visual field defects and their causes [1]

Visual field loss	Cause
Central scotoma	Lesions of the macula (e.g., macular degeneration, cystoid macular edema, inflammatory macular disease)
Ipsilateral monocular visual loss	Lesion in the optic nerve, leading to a complete visual field loss in the ipsilateral eye
Bitemporal hemianopia	Lesion of the optic chiasm or compression of the optic chiasm (e.g., pituitary adenomas, craniopharyngiomas)
Unilateral anopia	Lesion in the optic tract on the side of the anopia
Homonymous hemianopia	Lesion in the optic radiations on the contralateral side of the anopia
Homonymous hemianopia with macular sparing	Posterior cerebral artery stroke, leads to contralateral homonymous hemianopia
Cause of macular sparing	Dual blood supply via the middle cerebral artery and the posterior cerebral artery
Upper quadrantanopia	Lesion in the temporal lobe or a middle cerebral artery stroke in the contralateral side of the anopia
Lower quadrantanopia	Lesion in the parietal lobe or a stroke of the middle cerebral artery in the contralateral side of the anopia

which also carries the information from the temporal retina of the right eye. The right optic tract projects into the lateral geniculate nucleus of the right thalamus and is carried via the right optic radiation to the primary visual cortex located in the posterior occipital lobe within in the calcarine sulcus of the right hemisphere.

Note the difference between the left and right visual field. Table 9.1 shows a summary of common visual field defects and their causes.

9.4 Cranial Nerves

Figure 9.6 shows a schematic representation of the innervation target (either muscle or sensory organ) and termination of the optic nerve (CN II), oculomotor nerve (CN III), trochlear nerve (CN IV) , and abducens nerve (CN VI).

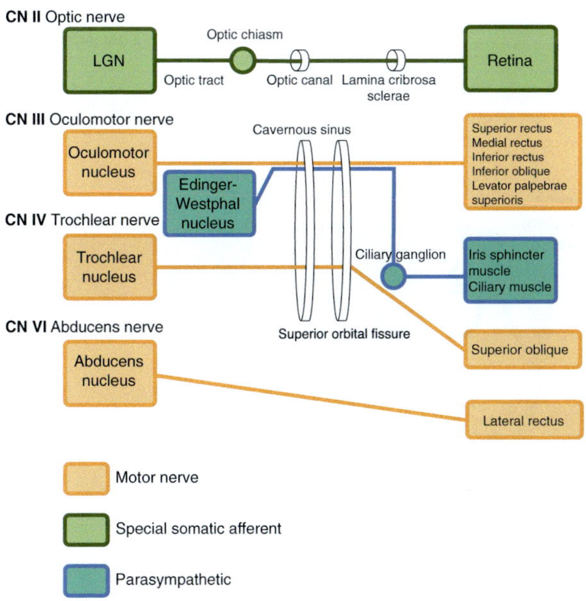

Fig. 9.6 The figure shows a schematic illustration of the cranial nerves associated with the eye, vision and the structures they innervate. The color-coding is explained in the legend

9.5 Pupil Reflexes

Changes in illumination detected by the photoreceptors on the retina trigger a nerve impulse that is transmitted by the optic nerves (CN II) via the optic chiasm and optic tracts

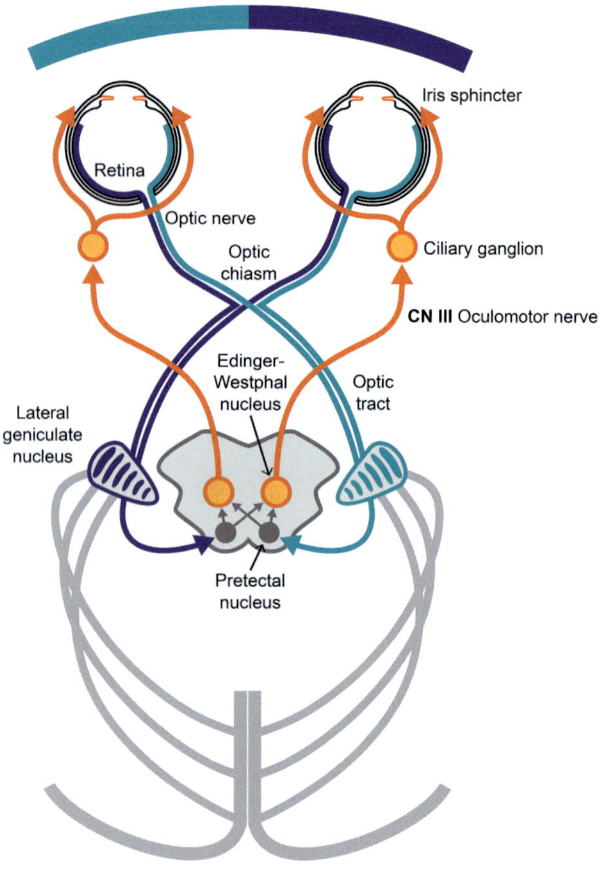

Fig. 9.7 The figure shows a schematic illustration of the pupil reflex pathway, the associated nerves, nuclei and ganglia and their anatomical relationship. Illustration: Samantha Strong (https://samstrongvision.com)

to the lateral geniculate nuclei. The lateral geniculate nuclei contain nerve fibres responsible for the pupil reflex which connect to the pretectal nuclei located in the midbrain (mesencephalon). From here, the information will be transmitted to equal parts to the Edinger-Westphal nuclei. The Edinger-Westphal nuclei send their information via the parasympathetic fibers of the oculomotor nerve (CN III) via the ciliary ganglion to the iris sphincter, which will lead to a dilatation (mydriasis) or constriction (myosis) of the iris, sphincter muscle (Fig. 9.7).

9.5.1 Swinging Light Test and Relative Afferent Pupillary Defect (RAPD)

Clinically, the swinging light test is utilized to detect a relative afferent pupil defect (RAPD). The purpose of this

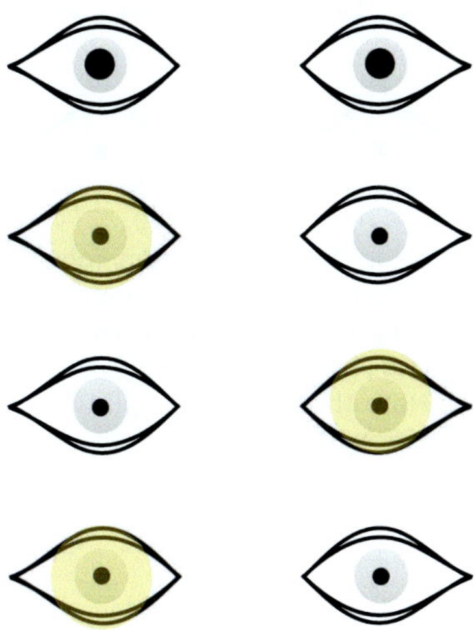

Fig. 9.8 The illustration shows a normal swinging light test without RAPD. The illumination of either eye elicits a normal and equal response (constriction) in the contralateral eye

test is to detect differences in the pupil response between the two eyes when light is shone on one eye at a time. This test can be useful to detect unilateral and asymmetrical diseases of the retina or optic nerve (CN II). Note, however, that the test only assesses optic nerve damage that occurs before the optic chiasm. Figures 9.8, 9.9, and 9.10 illustrate various common clinical scenarious and the corresponding pupil reactions.

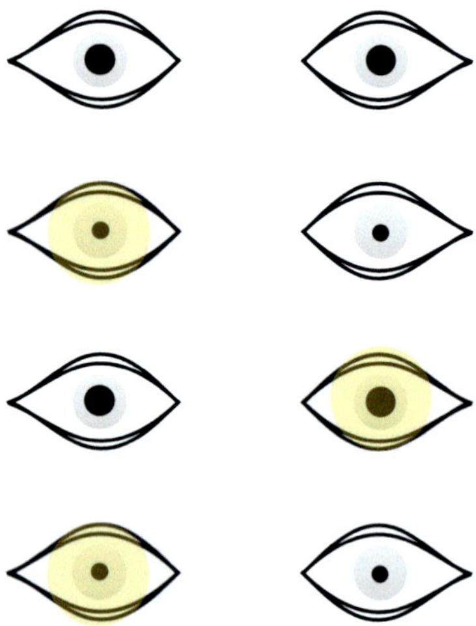

Fig. 9.9 The illustration shows a swinging light test with an RAPD in the left eye. The illumination of the normal right eye leads to a constriction of both pupils. However, when light is shone on the abnormal left eye (e.g., optic neuropathy), both pupils will dilate (less constriction). Note that the left pupil will dilate even when illuminated. Illumination of the normal right eye results in the constriction of both pupils

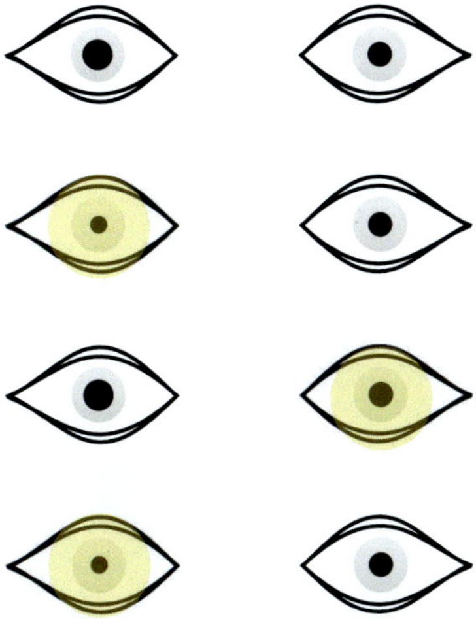

Fig. 9.10 The figure shows a swinging light test with an RAPD and a non-reactive left pupil. The illumination of the relatively normal right pupil leads to a constriction of only the right pupil. The illumination of the abnormal left pupil (fixed pupil and optic neuropathy) results in a dilatation of the right and constriction of the left pupil. Subsequent illumination of the right eye causes a constriction of the right pupil again. Under these circumstances, it is only necessary to observe the eye with the reactive pupil to identify RAPD

9.6 Extraocular Eye Muscles

Figure 9.11 shows an illustration of a left eye in the orbit and the extraocular muscles. The cranial nerves that innervate the extraocular muscles are summarized in Table 9.2. The main eye muscle actions are shown in Fig. 9.12. Figure 9.13 shows an illustration of the cardinal positions of gaze and the corresponding extraocular eye muscles (yoke muscles). Table 9.3 summarizes the primary, secondary and tertiary muscle actions.

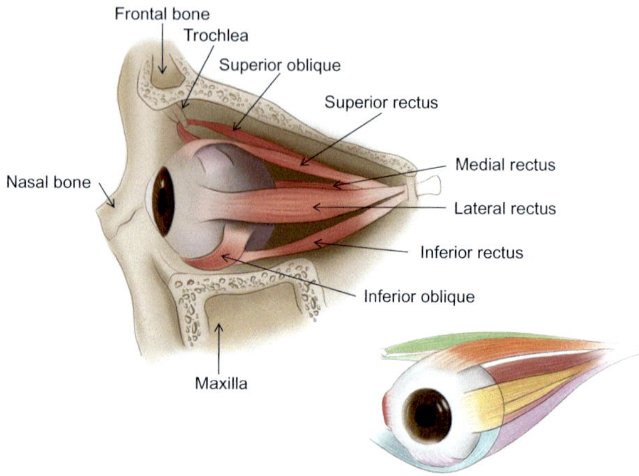

Fig. 9.11 The figure shows an illustration of the extraocular muscles of a left eye. The bottom figure shows a semi-transparent version of the muscles to visualize their relationship to each other. Illustrations: Sae Bom Ra

Table 9.2 Innervation of extraocular eye muscles

Muscle	Cranial nerve (CN)
Medial rectus	Oculomotor nerve (CN III)
Lateral rectus	Abducens nerve (CN VI)
Superior rectus	Oculomotor nerve (CN III)
Inferior rectus	Oculomotor nerve (CN III)
Superior oblique	Trochlear nerve (CN IV)
Inferior oblique	Oculomotor nerve (CN III)

9.6.1 Eye Muscle Actions

Table 9.3 summarizes the primary, secondary and tertiary muscle actions.

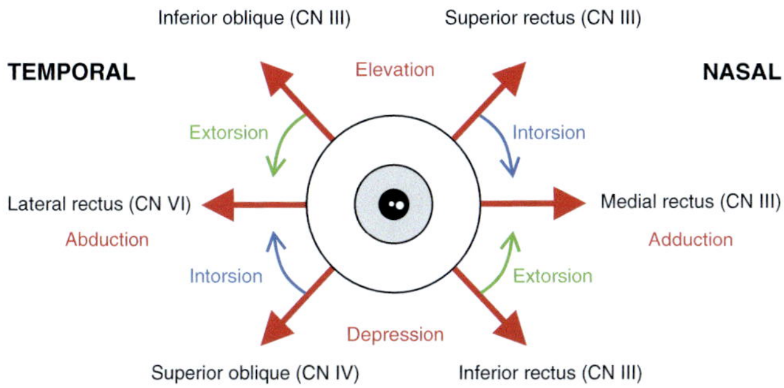

Fig. 9.12 Eye muscle movements

Table 9.3 Primary, secondary and tertiary muscle actions

Muscle	Primary action	Secondary action	Tertiary action
Medial rectus	Adduction	–	–
Lateral rectus	Abduction	–	–
Superior rectus	Elevation, maximum in abduction	Intorsion, maximum in adduction	Adduction, maximum in adduction
Inferior rectus	Depression, maximum in abduction	Extorsion, maximum in adduction	Adduction, maximum in adduction
Superior oblique	Intorsion, maximum in adduction	Depression, maximum in abdcution	Abduction, maximum in abduction
Inferior oblique	Extorsion, maximum in abduction	Elevation, maximum in adduction	Abduction, maximum in abduction

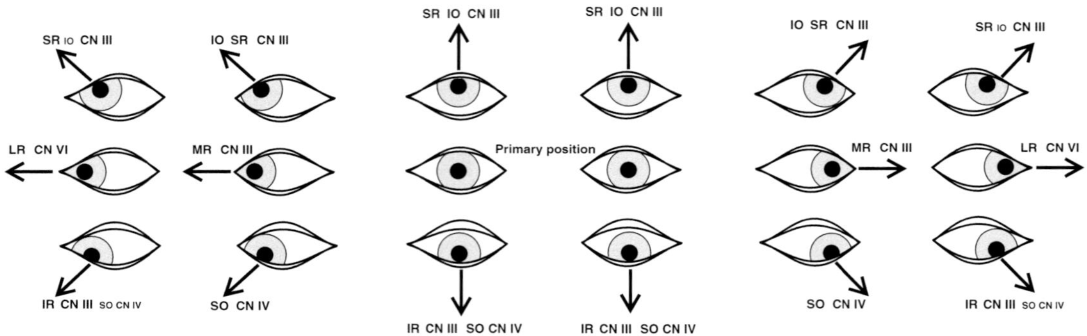

Fig. 9.13 The figure shows a schematic illustration of the cardinal positions of gaze and the corresponding extraocular eye muscles (yoke muscles). MR: Medial rectus, LR: Lateral rectus, SR: Superior rectus, IR: Inferior rectus, SO: Superior oblique, IO: Inferior oblique. A smaller font size indicates a smaller contribution. The corresponding cranial nerves are abbreviated as follows: CN III: Oculomotor nerve, CN IV: Trochlear nerve, CN VI: Abducens nerve

9.7 Binocular Vision

The following sections provide short definitions and illustrations of common binocular vision anomalies and how to identify them.

9.7.1 Heterotropia (Strabismus)

Heterotropia is a manifest misalignment of the eyes. One eye may turn inward (esotropia), outward (exotropia), upward (hypertropia), or downward (hypotropia). This can result in double vision (diplopia), poor depth perception, or suppression of the image from one eye to avoid diplopia. Figures 9.14 and 9.15 show how the eyes behave in an exotropia and esotropia using the cover/uncover test.

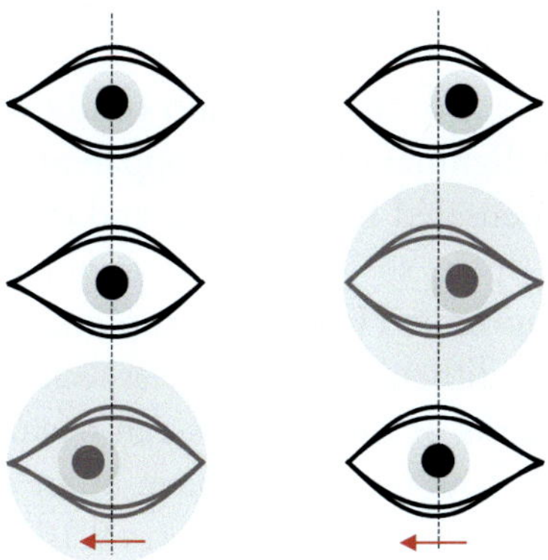

Fig. 9.14 The figure shows the eye movements during a cover/uncover test in the case of an exotropia in the left eye

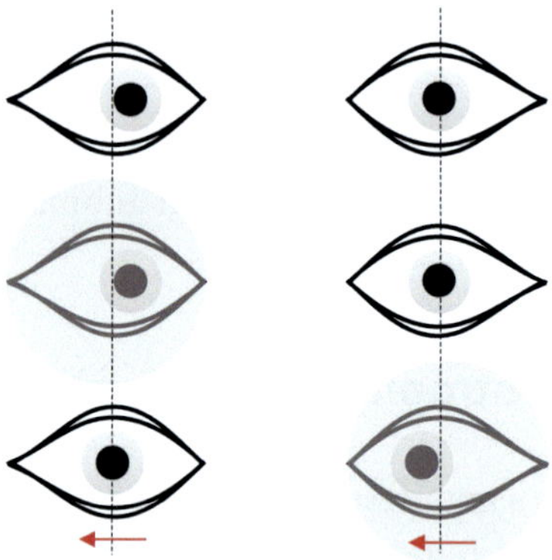

Fig. 9.15 The figure shows the eye movements during a cover/uncover test in the case of an esotropia in the right eye

9.7.2 Heterophoria (Latent Strabismus)

Heterophoria is a latent misalignment of the eyes. The eyes are capable to focus normally when both are open, but when one eye is covered (or under certain conditions, such as fatigue), the misalignment becomes apparent. Heterophorias are often compensated by the brain and eye muscles when both eyes are open, so the patient might not experience noticeable symptoms. However, symptoms like eye strain, headaches, and difficulty focusing, especially during prolonged visual tasks or under stress can occur. Figures 9.16 and 9.17 show how the eyes behave in an exophoria and esophoria using the cover test. Figures 9.18 and 9.19 show the eye movements during an alternate cover test in the presence of an exophoria and esophoria, respectively.

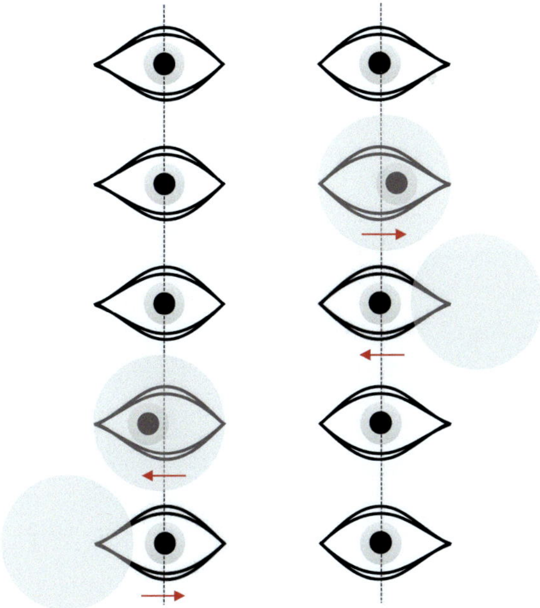

Fig. 9.16 The figure shows the eye movements during a cover test in the presence of an exophoria

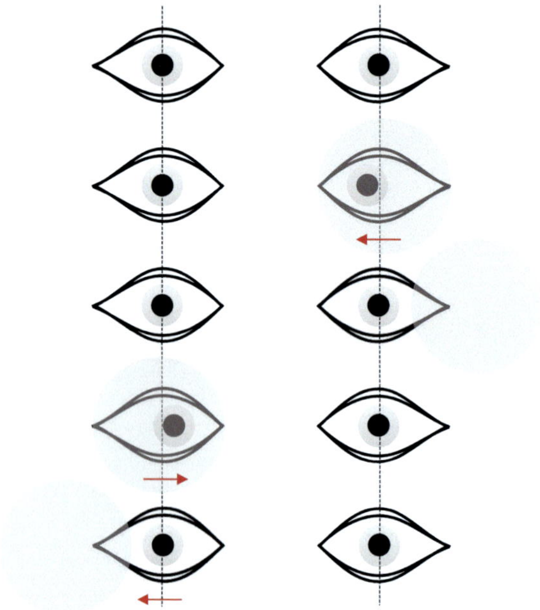

Fig. 9.17 The figure shows the eye movements during a cover test in the presence of an esophoria

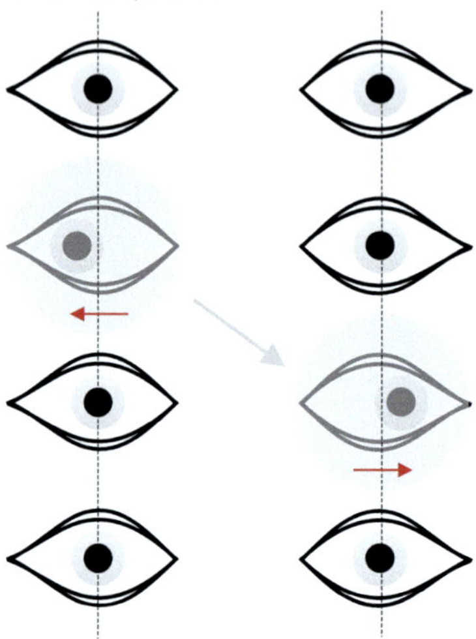

Fig. 9.18 The figure shows the eye movements during an alternate cover test in the presence of an exophoria

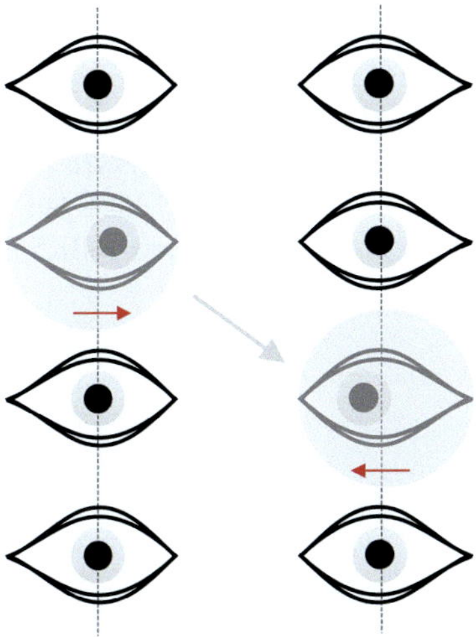

Fig. 9.19 The figure shows the eye movements during an alternate cover test in the presence of an esophoria

9.8 Further Reading

- Eperjesi F, Rundstrom MM. Practical binocular vision assessment. Elsevier Health Sciences; 2004.
- Evans BJ. Pickwell's binocular vision anomalies. Elsevier Health Sciences; 2021.
- Forrester JV, Dick AD, McMenamin PG, Roberts F, Pearlman E. The eye E-book: basic sciences in practice. Elsevier Health Sciences; 2015.
- Remington LA, Remington LA. Clinical anatomy and physiology of the visual system. Elsevier, 2012.
- Rowe FJ. Clinical orthoptics. John Wiley & Sons; 2012.
- Scheiman M, Wick B. Clinical management of binocular vision: heterophoric, accommodative, and eye movement disorders. Lippincott Williams & Wilkins; 2008.
- Waugh A, Grant A. Ross & Wilson Anatomy and physiology in health and illness E-book. Elsevier Health Sciences; 2014.

Reference

1. Gupta M, Ireland AC, Bordoni B. Neuroanatomy, visual pathway. [Updated 2022 Dec 19]. In: StatPearls [Internet]. Treasure Island (FL): StatPearls Publishing; 2024 Jan. Available from: https://www.ncbi.nlm.nih.gov/books/NBK553189/

10

Some Useful Numbers and Equations

10.1 Useful Numbers

Table 10.1 provides a summary of interesting numbers about the visual system.

Table 10.1 Useful numbers based on [1]

Structure/Property	Measurement	Source
Area of retina	1.094 mm^2	[2, 3]
Visual angle on retina	$1^\circ = 288\mu m$	[4]
Diameter of macula	3–4 mm	[5]
Diameter of central fovea	1.2–1.5 mm	[5]
Diameter of central rod-free area	250–750 μm	[5–8]
Diameter of central cone-free area	200–300 μm	[6–8]

(continued)

G. Schmidtmann, *Clinical Vision Science*, https://doi.org/10.1007/978-3-031-83321-2_10

Table 10.1 (continued)

Structure/Property	Measurement	Source
Density of cones in central fovea	96,900–238,000/mm^2	[8, 10, 11]
Number of cones in fovea	$200,000$	[10]
Density of cones in fovea	17,500/mm^2	[10]
Number of cones in the retina	$6,400,000$	[10]
Number of rods in the retina	110,000,000–125,000,000	[10]
Number of rods at $15°$	160,000/mm^2	[12]
Number of axons in the Optic nerve	564,776–1,200,000	[5, 13–15]
Number of neurons in primary visual cortex	$1.4x10^8 - 6.75x10^8$	[16, 17]
Visual field dimensions	Monocular: $160°$ (width) $\times 175°$ (height)	[18]
	Binocular: $200°$ (width) $\times 135°$ (height)	[18]
	Region of binocular overlap: $120°$ (width) $\times 135°$ (height)	[18]
Refractive power of Cornea	$43D$	[18]
Refractive power of Lens (without accommodation)	$20D$	[18]
Refractive power of eye	$63D$	[18]
Visible spectrum	370–730 nm	[18]

10.2 Descriptive Statistics

10.2.1 Arithmetic Mean

$$\bar{x} = \frac{1}{n}\left(\sum_{i=1}^{n} x_i\right) = \frac{x_1 + x_2 + \ldots + x_n}{n} \tag{10.1}$$

10.2.2 Geometric Mean

$$\bar{x} = \left(\prod_{i=1}^{n} x_i\right)^{1/n} = (x_1 \cdot x_2 \cdot \ldots \cdot x_n)^{1/n} \tag{10.2}$$

10.2.3 Measures of Spread

10.2.3.1 Variance

$$\sigma^2 = \frac{\sum_{i=1}^{n}(x_i - \bar{x})^2}{n - 1} \tag{10.3}$$

10.2.3.2 Standard Deviation

$$\sigma = \sqrt{\sigma^2} = \sqrt{\frac{\sum_{i=1}^{n}(x_i - \bar{x})^2}{n - 1}} \tag{10.4}$$

10.3 Further Reading

- Kolb H, Fernandez E, Nelson R. Webvision: the organization of the retina and visual system [Online]. Available: http://webvision.med.utah.edu/

References

1. Kolb H, Fernandez E, Nelson R. Webvision: the organization of the retina and visual system [Online]. Available: http://webvision.med.utah.edu/
2. Michels RG, Wilkinson CP, Rice TA. Retinal detachment. The C.V. Mosby Company; 1990. p. 17.
3. Penkhus J. The ora serrata and its anatomical variations. M.S. Thesis. Los Angeles: University of California; 1965.
4. Drasdo N, Fowler CW. Non-linear projection of the retinal image in a wide-angle schematic eye. Br J Ophthalmol. 1974;58:709–14.
5. Polyak SL. The retina. Chicago: University of Chicago Press; 1941.
6. Hendrickson AE, Youdelis C. The morphological development of the human fovea. Ophthalmology. 1984;91:603–12.
7. Yamada E. Some structural features of the fovea central is in the human retina. Arch Ophthalmol. 1969;82:151–9.
8. Ahnelt PK, Kolb H, Pflug R. Identification of a subtype of cone photoreceptor, likely to be blue sensitive, in the human retina. J Comp Neurol. 1987;255:18–34.
9. Ahnelt PK, Pflug R. Telodendrial contacts between foveolar cone pedicles in the human retina. Experientia. 1986;42:298–300.
10. Osterberg G. Topography of the layer of rods and cones in the human retina. Acta Ophthalmol Suppl. 1935;6:1–103.

11. Curcio CA, Sloan KR, Packer O, Hendrickson AE, Kalina RE. Distribution of cones in human and monkey retina: individual variability and radial asymmetry. Science. 1987;236:579–82.
12. Mariani AP, Kolb H, Nelson R. Dopamine-containing amacrine cells of rhesus monkey retina parallel rods in spatial distribution. Brain Res. 1984;322:1–7.
13. Bruesch SR, Arey LB. The number of myelinated and unmyelinated fibres in the optic nerve of vertebrates. J Comp Neurol. 1942;77:631.
14. Balazsi AG, Rootman J, Drance SM, Schulzer M, Douglas GR. The effect of age on the nerve fiber population of the human optic nerve. Am J Ophthalmol. 1984;97:760–6.
15. Quigley HA, Addicks EM, Green WR. Optic nerve damage inhuman glaucoma. III. Quantitative correlation of nerve fibre loss and visual defect in glaucoma ischemic neuropathy and toxic neuropathy. Arch Ophthalmol. 1982;100:135.
16. Leuba G, Kraftsik R. Changes in volume, surface estimate, three- dimensional shape and total number of neurons of the human primary visual cortex from midgestation until old age. Anatomy and embryology. 1994;190(4):351–66.
17. Miller DJ, Balaram P, Young NA, Kaas JH. Three counting methods agree on cell and neuron number in chimpanzee primary visual cortex. Front Neuroanat. 2014;8(36):1–11.
18. Wandell BA. Foundations of vision. Sunderland (MA): Sinauer Associates, Inc; 1965.

11

Exercise Solutions

This chapter contains the solutions to the exercises of each chapter. Please note that a lot of these exercises can be solved without the use of a calculator.

11.1 Basics

Note that all exercises below can be solved without the use of a calculator.

1. Convert the angle $\beta = 90°$ to radians.
   Solution

$$\beta_{Degree} = 90°$$

$$\beta_{Radians} = \frac{\beta_{Degree} \cdot \pi}{180°}$$

$$\beta_{Radians} = \frac{90° \cdot \pi}{180°}$$

$$\beta_{Radians} = \frac{1}{2} \cdot \pi = \frac{\pi}{2}$$

G. Schmidtmann, *Clinical Vision Science*,
https://doi.org/10.1007/978-3-031-83321-2_11

2. Convert the angle $\gamma = 2 \cdot \pi$ (radians) to degrees.
Solution

$$
\begin{aligned}
\gamma &= 2 \cdot \pi \\
\gamma_{Degree} &= \frac{\gamma_{Radians} \cdot 180^\circ}{\pi} \\
\gamma_{Degree} &= \frac{2 \cdot \pi \cdot 180^\circ}{\pi} \\
\gamma_{Degree} &= 2 \cdot 180^\circ = 360^\circ
\end{aligned}
$$

3. The hypothenuse of a right triangle has a lenght of $\sqrt{2}$, and the opposite has a length of 1. What is the length of the adjacent? Review Fig. 1.4 in Sect. 1.4.1.
Solution

$$
\begin{aligned}
a &= 1 \\
c &= \sqrt{2} \\
a^2 + b^2 &= c^2 \\
1^2 + b^2 &= \sqrt{2}^2 \\
1 + b^2 &= 2 \\
b^2 &= 2 - 1 = 1 \\
b &= \sqrt{1} = 1
\end{aligned}
$$

The opposite has a length of 1.

4. What is the solution of $log_{10}10,000$?
   Solution
   Remember the relationship between exponentiations and logarithms covered in Sect. 1.5.

$$\log_{10} 10,000$$
$$10^x = 10,000$$
$$x = 4$$
$$\log_{10} 10,000 = 4$$

5. Rearrange $x = 2 \cdot e^{4y^2}$ to make y the subject.
   Solution

$$x = 2 \cdot e^{4y^2}$$
$$\frac{x}{2} = e^{4y^2}$$
$$\ln\left(\frac{x}{2}\right) = 4y^2$$
$$\frac{1}{4}\ln\left(\frac{x}{2}\right) = y^2$$
$$y = \pm\sqrt{\frac{1}{4}\ln\left(\frac{x}{2}\right)}$$

6. The Force F is calculated according to the equation $F = m \cdot a$, where m is the mass measured in kg and a is the acceleration measured in $^m/_{s^2}$. Derive the SI unit of the Force F? Hint: Newton is not the answer we are looking for!

Solution

$$F = m \cdot a$$

Replace m and a with their SI units.

$$F = \left[kg \cdot \frac{m}{s^2}\right]$$

See Table 1.4 in Sect. 1.8.

11.2 Physical Optics

1. Calculate the wavelength of light traveling with the speed of light (assuming $c = 3 \cdot 10^5 {km}/{s}$) and a frequency of $10^{12}\ Hz$.
   Solution

$$c = 3 \cdot 10^5 {km}/{s} = 3 \cdot 10^8 {m}/{s}$$
$$f = 10^{12} {1}/{s}$$
$$f = \frac{c}{\lambda}$$
$$\lambda = \frac{c}{f}$$
$$\lambda = \frac{3 \cdot 10^8\ ms}{10^{12}\ s}$$
$$\lambda = 3 \cdot 10^{-4}\ m$$

2. A light ray is traveling into a block of Crown Glass ($n = 1.523$) with a width of $4\ cm$ surrounded by air. The angle of incidence is 30°. Calculate the angle of refraction?

Solution

$$\sin\theta_1 \cdot n_1 = \sin\theta_2 \cdot n_2$$
$$\theta_2 = \sin^{-1}\left(\frac{n_1 \cdot \sin\theta_1}{n_2}\right)$$
$$\theta_2 = \sin^{-1}\left(\frac{1 \cdot \sin 30^\circ}{1.523}\right) = 19.17^\circ$$

3. Derive the equation for the lateral deplacement s (see Eq. 2.8 in Sect. 2.2.3).
   Solution

$$\cos\theta_2 = \frac{t}{h}$$
$$h = \frac{t}{\cos\theta_2}$$
$$\delta = \theta_1 - \theta_2$$
$$\sin\delta = \frac{s}{h}$$
$$s = \frac{\sin\delta}{h}$$
$$s = \frac{t \cdot \sin(\theta_1 - \theta_2)}{\cos\theta_2}$$

4. Calculate the angle of deviation when light is incident at 40° on the surface of a block of glass with a refractive index of $n = 1.5$?

Solution

$$
\begin{aligned}
sin\theta_1 \cdot n &= \sin\theta_2 \cdot n' \\
\theta_2 &= \sin^{-1}\left(\frac{n \cdot \sin\theta_1}{n'}\right) \\
\theta_2 &= \sin^{-1}\left(\frac{1 \cdot \sin 40^\circ}{1.5}\right) \\
\theta_2 &= 25.4^\circ
\end{aligned}
$$

5. What is the lateral displacement s if a ray of light hits a block of glass with a refractive index of $n = 1.523$ and a width of $t = 2\,cm$ with angle of incidence of 30°?

Solution
Please see Fig. 2.2.

$$
\begin{aligned}
\theta_1 &= 30^\circ \\
\sin\theta_2 &= \frac{n \sin\theta_1}{n'} \\
\theta_2 &= \sin^{-1}\left(\frac{\sin 30^\circ}{1.523}\right) \\
\theta_2 &= 19.1^\circ \\
\delta &= \theta_1 - \theta_2 \\
\delta &= 30^\circ - 19.1^\circ = 10.9^\circ \\
h &= \frac{t}{\cos\theta_2} \\
h &= \frac{0.02m}{\cos 19.1^\circ} \\
h &= 0.0212m \\
s &= h \cdot \sin\delta \\
s &= 0.0212m \cdot \sin 10.9^\circ \\
s &= 0.004m = 0.4cm
\end{aligned}
$$

Alternatively, you could use Eq. 2.8. First, we must calculate the angle of refraction θ_2 (see Eq. 2.7).

$$\theta_2 = \sin^{-1}\left(\frac{n \cdot \sin\theta_1}{n'}\right)$$
$$\theta_2 = \sin^{-1}\left(\frac{\sin 30^\circ}{1.523}\right)$$
$$\theta_2 = 19.1^\circ$$

Now we use Eq. 2.8 to calculate the lateral displacement s.

$$s = \frac{t \cdot \sin(\theta_1 - \theta_2)}{\cos\theta_2}$$
$$s = \frac{0.02m \cdot \sin(30^\circ - 19.1^\circ)}{\cos 19.1^\circ}$$
$$s = 0.004\ m = 0.4\ cm$$

6. An object in air is located 100 mm away from a surface separating air and glass ($n = 1.5$). The image is formed 10 cm within the glass. What is the power of the surface?

Solution

$$L = \frac{1}{l}$$
$$L = \frac{1}{-0.1m}$$
$$L = -10D$$
$$L' = \frac{n'}{l'}$$
$$L' = \frac{1.5}{0.1m}$$
$$L' = 15D$$
$$F = L' - L$$
$$F = 15D + 10D = 25D$$

7. A prism made of glass ($n = 1.523$) and an apical angle of $\alpha = 30°$ is submerged in water ($n = 1.333$). The angle of incidence $\theta = 40°$. Calculate the total angle of deviation?

Solution

Please see Fig. 2.4.

$$\sin\theta_2 = \frac{n \sin\theta_1}{n'}$$
$$\theta_2 = \sin^{-1}\left(\frac{n \cdot \sin\theta_1}{n'}\right)$$
$$\theta_2 = \sin^{-1}\left(\frac{1.333 \cdot \sin 40°}{1.523}\right)$$
$$\theta_2 = 34.24°$$
$$\delta_1 = \theta_1 - \theta_2$$
$$\delta_1 = 40° - 34.24° = 5.76°$$

$$\alpha = \theta_2 - \theta_1$$
$$\theta_3 = \alpha - \theta_2$$
$$\theta_3 = 40^\circ - 34.24^\circ$$
$$\theta_3 = 5.76^\circ$$
$$\sin\theta_3 \cdot n = \sin\theta_4 \cdot n'$$
$$\theta_4 = \sin^{-1}\left(\frac{n \cdot \sin\theta_3}{n'}\right)$$
$$\theta_4 = \sin^{-1}\left(\frac{1.523 \cdot \sin 5.76^\circ}{1.333}\right)$$
$$\theta_4 = 6.58^\circ$$
$$\delta_2 = \theta_3 - \theta_4$$
$$\delta_2 = 5.76^\circ - 6.58^\circ$$
$$\delta_2 = -0.82^\circ$$
$$\delta_3 = \delta_1 + \delta_2$$
$$\delta_3 = 5.76^\circ - 0.82^\circ = 4.94^\circ$$

8. What is the critical angle for total internal reflection to occur within a block of transparent plastic ($n' = 1.4$) surrounded by air?
Solution

$$\sin\theta_c = \frac{n}{n'}$$
$$\theta_c = \sin^{-1}\left(\frac{n}{n'}\right)$$
$$\theta_c = \sin^{-1}\left(\frac{1}{1.4}\right)$$
$$\theta_c = 45.6^\circ$$

9. A lens system is composed of two lenses, where lens 1 has a refractive power $F_1 = -2D$ and lens 2 a refractive power $F_2 = -1$. The distance between the two lenses is $d = 3\,cm$. An object is located 25 cm in front of lens. Calculate the position of the resulting image with respect to lens 2.

Solution

$$L_1 = \frac{1}{l}$$

$$L_1 = \frac{1}{-0.25\ m} = -4D$$

$$L_1' = F_1 + L_1$$

$$L_1' = -2D - 4D = -6D$$

$$l_1' = \frac{1}{L_1'}$$

$$l_1' = \frac{1}{-6D} = -0.1667\ m$$

$$l_2 = l' - d$$

$$l_2 = -0.1667\ m - 0.03\ m = -0.1967\ m$$

$$L_2 = \frac{1}{l_2}$$

$$L_2 = \frac{1}{-0.1967\ m} = -5.084D$$

$$L_2' = F_2 + L_2$$

$$L_2' = -1 - 5.084D = -6.084D$$

$$l_2' = \frac{1}{-6.084D} = -0.164\ m$$

The image is located 16.4 cm in front of lens 2.

10. A lens system is made up of a $+20.00D$ lens and a $+30.00D$ lens separated by 10 cm. The lenses are surrounded by air. Assume a thick lens with a refractive index $n = 1.523$. What is the back vertex power of the lens system? Find the solution by using both, the step-along method and the formula.
Solution

$$F_1 = +20D$$
$$F_2 = +30D$$
$$d = 10cm = 0.1m$$
$$n = 1$$
$$n' = 1.523$$

Step-along Method
We are interested in the Back Vertex Power (BVP, F'_v), hence we assume a vergence in of $L = 0D$.

$$L' = F_1 + L$$
$$L' = +20D + 0 = +20D$$
$$L' = \frac{n}{l'}$$
$$l' = \frac{1.523}{+20D} = 0.07615\ m$$
$$l_2 = l' - d$$
$$l_2 = 0.07615\ m - 0.1\ m = -0.02385\ m$$
$$L_2 = \frac{n'}{l_2}$$
$$L_2 = \frac{1.523}{-0.02385m} = -63.86D$$

$$L_2' = F_2 + L_2$$
$$L_2' = +30D - 63.86D = -33.86D$$
$$L_2' = F_v' = -33.86D$$

Formula

$$F_v' = \frac{F_1 + F_2 - (\frac{d}{n'}) \cdot F_1 \cdot F_2}{1 - (\frac{d}{n'}) \cdot F_1}$$
$$F_v' = \frac{+20 + 30 - (\frac{0.1}{1.523}) \cdot 20 \cdot 30}{1 - (\frac{0.1}{1.523}) \cdot 20}$$
$$F_v' = -33.86D$$

11.3 Visual Optics

1. Calculate the change in back vertex power required for specular refraction of $-7\,D$ when the back vertex distance is changed from $15\,mm$ to $5\,mm$.
Solution

$$F_{v1}' = -7D$$
$$d_1 = 0.015\ m$$
$$d_2 = 0.005\ m$$
$$F_{v2}' = \frac{F_{v1}'}{1 + (d_2 - d_1) \cdot F_{v1}'}$$
$$F_{v2}' = \frac{-7D}{1 + (0.005m - 0.015m) \cdot -7D}$$

$$F'_{v2} = 6.54D$$

2. A myopic patient with a prescription of $-5.00D$ is corrected for the distance with a spectacle lens placed at 10 mm in front of the eye. Calculate the accommodation (A) required when viewing an object at 30 cm in front of the spectacle lens. If this eye was then corrected with a contact lens, how much accommodation is required when viewing the same object?

Solution

$$k = \frac{n}{K}$$

$$k = \frac{1}{-5D} = -0.2\ m$$

$$f'_{sp} = k + d$$

$$f'_{sp} = -0.2m + 0.01\ m = -0.21\ m$$

$$F'_{sp} = \frac{n}{f'_{sp}}$$

$$F'_{sp} = \frac{1}{-0.21m} = -4.76D$$

$$L' = L + F'_{sp} = \frac{1}{l_{sp}} + F'_{sp}$$

$$L' = \frac{1}{-0.3m} + (-4.76D) = -8.09D$$

$$l' = \frac{1}{L'} = \frac{1}{-8.09D} = -0.124\ m$$

$$l_2 = l' - d$$

$$l_2 = -0.124\ m - 0.01\ m = -0.134\ m$$

$$L_2 = \frac{1}{l_2}$$

$$L_2 = \frac{1}{-0.134m} = -7.49D$$

$$A_{sp} = K - L_2$$
$$A_{sp} = -5D - (-7.49D) = 2.49D$$

Correction with contact lens.

$$l_{cl} = -0.3m - 0.01m = -0.31m$$
$$L_{cl} = \frac{1}{l_{cl}}$$
$$L_{cl} = \frac{1}{l_{-0.31m}} = -3.23D$$
$$A_{cl} = (-L_{cl}) = 3.23D$$

11.4 Ophthalmic Lenses

1. What is the sphero-cylindrical power for the following combination of obliquely crossed cylinders?
   Lens A: $-3.50/-4.00 \times 45°$
   Lens B: $-2.50/-1.50 \times 90°$
   Use the astigmatic decomposition method.
   Solution
   Lens A

$$C_0 = C_1 \cdot cos(2 \cdot \theta)$$
$$C_0 = -4.00D \cdot cos(2 \cdot 45°)$$
$$C_0 = 0D$$
$$C_{45} = C_1 \cdot sin(2 \cdot cyl_1)$$
$$C_{45} = -4.00D \cdot sin(2 \cdot 45°)$$
$$C_{45} = -4.00D$$

$$M_1 = S_1 + \frac{C_1}{2}$$
$$M_1 = -3.50D + \frac{-4.00D}{2}$$
$$M_1 = -5.50D$$

Lens B

$$C_0 = C_2 \cdot cos(2 \cdot \theta)$$
$$C_0 = -1.50D \cdot cos(2 \cdot 90°)$$
$$C_0 = 1.50D$$
$$C_{45} = C_1 \cdot sin(2 \cdot cyl_1)$$
$$C_{45} = -1.50D \cdot sin(2 \cdot 90°)$$
$$C_{45} = 0D$$
$$M_1 = S_1 + \frac{C_1}{2}$$
$$M_1 = -2.50D + \frac{-1.50D}{2}$$
$$M_1 = -3.25D$$

$$C_R = \pm\sqrt{\sum C_0^2 + \sum C_{45}^2}$$
$$C_R = \pm\sqrt{1.50D^2 + 4.00D^2}$$
$$C_R = -4.27D$$

$$S = \sum M - \left(\frac{C_R}{2}\right)$$
$$S = -8.75D - \frac{-4.27D}{2}$$
$$S = -6.615D$$

$$\tan\theta = \frac{C_R - \sum C_0}{\sum C_{45}}$$
$$\tan\theta = 1.1443$$
$$\theta = 55.27^\circ$$

$$-6.615/-4.27 \times 55.27 \rightarrow -6.50/-4.25 \times 55$$

2. What is the sphero-cylindrical power for the following combination of obliquely crossed cylinders?
   Lens A: $-1.00/-2.00 \times 20^\circ$
   Lens B: $-2.50/-3.00 \times 80^\circ$
   Use the calculation method (Table 11.1).
   Solution

$$\alpha = \theta_{cyl_2} - \theta_{cyl_1}$$
$$\alpha = 80^\circ - 20^\circ = 60^\circ$$
$$\gamma = \frac{atan\left(\frac{|C_2| sin2\alpha}{|C_1| + |C_2| cos2\alpha}\right)}{2}$$
$$\gamma = \frac{atan\left(\frac{|-3.00D| sin2 \cdot 60^\circ}{|-2.00D| + |-3.00D| cos2 \cdot 60^\circ}\right)}{2}$$
$$\gamma = 39.6^\circ$$
$$\theta_{cyl} = \gamma + \theta_{cyl_1}$$
$$\theta_{cyl} = 39.6^\circ + 20^\circ = 59.6^\circ$$
$$S = C_1 \cdot sin(\gamma)^2 + C_2 \cdot sin(\alpha - \gamma)^2$$
$$S = -2.00D \cdot sin(39.6^\circ)^2 - 3.00D \cdot sin(60^\circ - 39.6^\circ)^2$$

Table 11.1 Astigmatic decomposition

	M	C_0	C_{45}
Lens 1	$-5.50D$	$0D$	$-4.00D$
Lens 2	$-3.25D$	$1.50D$	0
$\sum$	$-8.75D$	$1.50D$	$-4.00D$

$$S = -1.18D$$
$$C_R = C_1 + C_2 - 2S$$
$$C_R = -2.00D - 3.00D - (2 \cdot -1.18D)$$
$$C_R = -2.64D$$
$$S_{total} = S + S_1 + S_2$$
$$S_{total} = -1.18D - 1.00D - 2.500D$$
$$S_{total} = -4.68D$$

$$-4.68/-2.64 \times 60 \rightarrow -4.75/-2.75 \times 60$$

11.5 Optical Instruments

1. Calculate the size of the retinal image of an object with a height of 30 cm located at a distance of 1 m away from a schematic reduced eye with an axial length of 22 mm.
   Solution

$$m = \frac{h'}{h} = \frac{L}{L'}$$
$$L = \frac{n}{l}$$
$$L = \frac{1}{-1m} = -1D$$
$$L' = \frac{n'}{l'}$$
$$L' = \frac{4/3}{0.022\,m} = 60.45D$$
$$m = \frac{L}{L'}$$

$$m = \frac{-1D}{60.45D} = -0.0165$$
$$h' = h \cdot m$$
$$h' = 0.3m \cdot (-0.0165) = -0.005\ m = -5\ mm$$

2. Calculate the size of the retinal image in an eye which has been corrected with a $-12.00D$ spectacle lens positioned at a distance of 10 mm in front of the eye, if the size of the uncorrected retinal image is 0.5 mm? Assume a thin lens.
Solution

$$M_s = \frac{1}{1 - (d \cdot F_{sp})}$$
$$M_s = \frac{1}{1 - (0.01m \cdot -12.00D)} = 1.12$$
$$M_s = \frac{h'_{cc}}{h'_{sc}}$$
$$h'_{cc} = M_s \cdot h'_{sc}$$
$$h'_{cc} = 1.12 \cdot 0.5\ mm = 0.56\ mm$$

11.6 Photometry

1. Calculate the solid angle (ω) subtended at the center of a sphere with a diameter (d) of 1 m, by an area of 2.5 m^2 on the surface of the sphere.
Solution

$$r = radius$$

$$r = \frac{d}{2}$$

$$r = \frac{1m}{2} = 0.5m$$

$$\omega = \frac{A}{r^2}$$

$$\omega = \frac{2.5m^2}{(0.5m)^2} = 10sr$$

2. Calculate the illumination on a horizontal surface located 2 m directly below a point source of light with the intensity of 200cd.
Solution

$$E_v = \frac{I_v}{r^2}$$

$$E_v = \frac{200cd}{(2m)^2} = 50lux$$

3. A point light source with the intensity of 200cd is positioned at a distance of 2 m from a horizontal surface. Calculate the illumination on that surface for a point that is located 1 m away (Fig. 11.1).
Solution

$$r^2 = x^2 + h^2$$

$$r = \sqrt{(1m)^2 + (2m)^2} = \sqrt{5}m$$

$$\theta = \cos^{-1}\left(\frac{h}{r}\right)$$

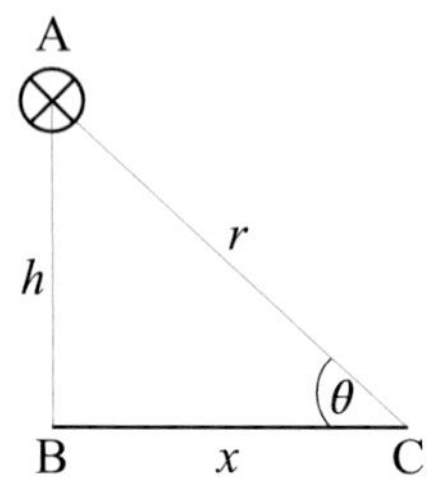

Fig. 11.1 Illustration of illumination scenario (not to scale; $h = 2\,m, x = 1\,m$)

$$\theta = \cos^{-1}\left(\frac{2m}{\sqrt{5}m}\right) = 26.57^\circ$$

$$E_v = \frac{I_v}{r^2} \cdot \cos\theta$$

$$E_v = \frac{200cd}{(\sqrt{5}m)^2} \cdot \cos 26.57^\circ = 35.76lux$$

11.7 Testing Visual Functions

1. A Tumbling E is presented at a distance of $d = 6\,m$. A patient achieves a visual acuity of $-0.1 log$MAR.

   a. What is the size of a single stroke (stroke width, S_w) of the Tumbling E?

$$\text{MAR} = 10^{log\text{MAR}}$$

$$\text{MAR} = 10^{-0.1} = 0.7943'$$

$$\text{MAR} = \frac{0.7943'}{60^\circ} = 0.013^\circ$$

$$S_w = \tan(\text{MAR}) \cdot d$$

$$S_w = \tan 0.013^\circ \cdot 6\,m = 1.36 \cdot 10^{-3}\,m = 1.36\,mm$$

b. What is the overall size S of the Tumbling E in mm?

$$S = S_w \cdot 5$$
$$S = 1.36\ mm \cdot 5 = 6.8\ mm$$

2. Convert the minimum angle of resolution MAR $= 0.63'$ into a Snellen fraction, assuming a viewing distance of 6 m.

Solution

$$logMAR = \log_{10} \text{MAR}$$
$$\log_{10} 0.63' = -0.20$$
$$logMAR = \log_{10} S_n - \log_{10} S_d$$
$$\log_{10} S_n = logMAR + \log_{10} S_d$$
$$\log_{10} S_n = -0.20 + \log_{10} 6 = 0.58$$
$$S_n = 10^{0.58} = 3.79 \approx 3.80$$
$$\text{Snellen} = \frac{6}{3.80}$$

Index

G. Schmidtmann, *Clinical Vision Science*,
https://doi.org/10.1007/978-3-031-83321-2

MIX
Papier aus verantwortungsvollen Quellen
Paper from responsible sources
FSC® C105338

If you have any concerns about our products,
you can contact us on
ProductSafety@springernature.com

In case Publisher is established outside the EU,
the EU authorized representative is:
Springer Nature Customer Service Center GmbH
Europaplatz 3, 69115 Heidelberg, Germany

Printed by Libri Plureos GmbH
in Hamburg, Germany